AF419826

Holistic
Psychotherapy
from a
Post-Materialist
Perspective

Holistic
Psychotherapy from a Post-Materialist Perspective

Margaret Arnd-Caddigan

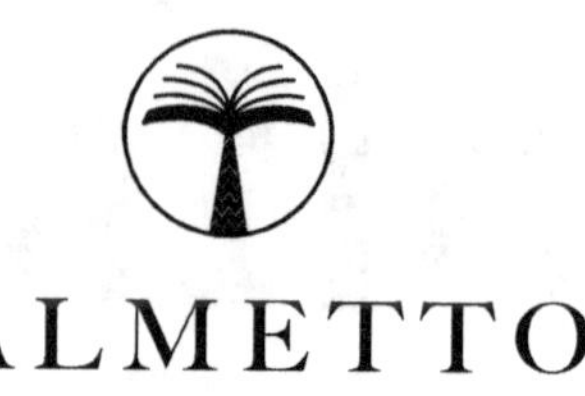

Charleston, SC
www.PalmettoPublishing.com

© 2024 by Margaret Arnd-Caddigan
All rights reserved.

This book or any portion thereof may not be reproduced or used in any manner whatsoever without the express written permission of the publisher except for the use of brief quotations in a book review.

Paperback ISBN: 979-8-8229-4166-3
eBook: 979-8-8229-4167-0

Contents

Preface

A colleague of mine once said that knowledge is like the water in an old-fashioned ice cube tray: the water is a single body—it's one thing—until we place a separator in it. Then we freeze it into disconnected chunks that we call distinct disciplines. That's the way I see knowledge, and that's the way I see people. In order to help anyone, we have to let them thaw and remove the partitions so that they can experience their fundamental unity. That's holistic therapy in a nutshell.

I operate from the premise that in mental health we have paid too much attention to the body to the exclusion of the mind. In response, I practice what I have come to call a mind-centered approach. "But wait," you may ask, "how is *mind*-centered holistic? Doesn't that ignore all of the other aspects of humanity?" Indeed, mind-centered means we center the mind. But centering the mind does not mean ignoring or minimizing all of our other dimensions. Our minds are inextricably involved in every facet of our being. Psyche, which means mind, also means spirit. Our minds and our spirituality are one. Our minds are inseparable from social relations. Our minds and our bodies are two sides of a single coin. Our minds are associated with a phenomenon we call energy. But today, our mind has been reduced to a side effect of neurochemical processes. We have been taught that our minds are weak and fallible. They lead us away from the truth. It is our bodies—our eyes, our ears, and the rest of our senses but mostly our brains—that are the royal road to understanding Reality. I call my way of doing therapy "mind-centered" as a way to call attention to the fact that the time has come to return to an appreciation of how important our minds are to our well-being. Our minds require as much attention as our bodies in understanding why people suffer and how they can thrive.

This book was written for every therapist who chafed at seeing their clients as machines in meat suits, for every therapist who was unable to keep a client bound to a manual. It was written for every therapist who knows there is more to a good life than symptom reduction. It was written for every therapist who has always known that a good society can only be created by healthy people. That's holism. It's all connected; we're all connected.

I have conducted, researched, taught, and supervised psychotherapy for decades. I have taught practice courses and theory courses. What I've learned from my research is that each seasoned therapist conducts their own brand of therapy. Integration of practices is perhaps more widespread than some researchers and professors would like us to believe. But what I heard in my research on clinical intuition is that some therapists integrate more than therapy schools. They integrate all of the knowledge and experience they have in regard to what it means to be human and what it means to live a good life. They consume the humanities; they use philosophy, religion and spirituality, sociology, and so on in the work they do with their clients. It is time to bring this way of doing therapy out of the shadows and support therapists who wish to engage in their art from a more holistic perspective. My hope is that this book is one step in that journey.

Of course, this work is the culmination of many connections. It could not exist without the many people who have supported me through the process—all of the clients, supervisees, and teachers who have poured water into my tray, all of the colleagues and friends who listened patiently as I hashed out awkward half-formed ideas and far-out theories. Thank you, Dayna Farrington and Amber Perry for reading a rough first draft and giving me valuable feedback. I thank the members of the Greenville Psychoanalytic Study Group who gave me room to bring my woo-woo ideas into the conversation every month. David Caddigan gave the manuscript a close reading and offered invaluable suggestions. And my family—I cannot begin to address the appreciation I have for everything they have given me.

Chapter One

Introduction

If you consume any kind of media at all, you've probably been inundated by concerns about the mental health crisis. If you have been practicing psychotherapy for a while, you know how many people are seeking services. People are hurting, and there's good reason to believe that psychotherapy can help. After all, there is a body of research that has demonstrated that people who engage in psychotherapy usually get better (Wampold 2010). But what we mean when we decry the poor state of mental health and what we mean when we say people are "better" are issues of some controversy.

Many writers and researchers have pointed to the rise of the medical model in mental health as an impairment to well-being that must be overcome (Wampold 2010). After all, is the issue that needs to be resolved really an illness? Is it a distinct syndrome with clearly identifiable etiology and a unique set of symptoms? No, it's not. Is it a disease of the brain? There are some post-materialist psychologists and other scholars who resoundingly say no. They assert that mind is not reducible to the brain or more broadly to neurochemical processes or the body or anything material (Arnd-Caddigan 2021).

As early as the 1970s, Jerome Frank had identified the kinds of suffering psychotherapists help resolve as "demoralization" (quoted in

Duncan 2010, 3-22). The way to relieve this demoralization is through healing—healing that is common to "psychotherapy, group and family therapies, inpatient treatment, drug therapy, medicine, religiomagical healing in nonindustrialized societies, cults, and revivals." As a healing method, Frank identified the panoply of therapies as "a single entity" (quoted in Duncan 2010, p. 7).

We recognize in Frank's work the precursor of today's holistic therapies. As we will see, holistic therapy is not a single manualized treatment but a logic that unites a multitude of healing approaches to bring about well-being. In most cases, the healing is targeted to the sense of self, or simply self. Self is an aspect of mind, and so in healing the self, we are helping people heal their minds.

In the next chapter, we will look at the history of Western ideas about the nature of mind. Thoughts about mind run from the birth of science, the incorporation of the scientific method and worldview into medicine, and the medicalization of mental suffering. We will see how science—or more precisely scientism—has been normalized to the degree that we take it for granted as the explanation for everything, including mind and mental suffering. But this trend is being challenged by a number of scientists, psychologists, and philosophers. Many reasonable, educated thinkers are asserting that the dominant orienting assumption about mind—that it is a side effect of activity of the brain or neurochemical processes—is neither accurate nor helpful in helping people who are suffering.

Chapter three is an overview of some of the popular conceptualizations of holistic therapy. I hope that as we review the various perspectives and practices, we can begin to construct a sense of how we might wish to define holistic therapy. I will argue that some of the treatment approaches that are termed "holistic" in the popular literature are not in fact inclusive enough to warrant the label. Some continue the bio-reductionist tradition. Some include spirituality and spiritual practices in their work. I argue that this is important but does not constitute a comprehensive holistic approach. There are many approaches which include considerations beyond the mind and the body. Many include mind, body, and spirituality in their models. For some, energy is an important component in treatment. Thompson (2019, 2020, 64-71) has asserted that we must include the social nature of mind in our treatment of mental suffering. Edge (2011) has suggested that a mixture of elements is not sufficient for an approach to be holistic: there must be an underlying or unifying reason or logic that ties the collection of disciplines, therapy schools, and techniques together.

There are two highly developed approaches to therapy that include all of these elements in varying degrees. These are Psychosynthesis and Integral Therapy. In chapters four and five, I describe these two approaches in some detail. We will see that Integral Therapy has two different expressions: that of Cortright and that of Wilber/Forman. They are both based on a unifying worldview that combines Eastern and Western perspectives regarding what it means to be human and what it means to function optimally. They also differ in important ways. Perhaps the chief area of divergence is the degree to which human development is viewed as a normative, linear process, and clients are understood in terms of where they are located in a complicated matrix of developmental achievements and deficits.

In chapter six, I illustrate the way that I have combined the elements of holistic therapy under the aegis of a unifying paradigm. I call my resulting approach to psychotherapy a mind-centered depth approach. This chapter represents a continuation of the work I began in my book *Intuition in Therapy Practice: A Mind-Centered Approach for Healing* (2021). In chapter six, I look at theoretical elements of a mind-centered therapy. The cornerstone of this approach is an understanding of the self as the experiencer of experience. What this means is that if we are going to help people change their minds, we work to help them change their sense of self. I break down components that are important in this work as well as acknowledge the role of developmental models, the importance of consciousness (and the unconscious), meaning, and the role of emotions as Thompson emphasized.

In chapter seven, I look at my mind-centered approach on a more practical level. Like Frank, I see healing as a single category. Based on the research into healing, I call for holistic therapists to focus on connection, intention, and attention as part of a reflective practice aimed at exploring consciousness and ultimately helping our clients change their minds. In this process, the therapist will be mindful of the common factors and engage in the judicious use of interpretation. I included three case examples at the end of the chapter to show how I use various techniques toward the objectives laid out in chapter six.

We see that, in the holistic psychotherapy movement, we are coming back to the work of Frank and others who understood psychotherapy to be a healing practice. It is a practice that stands in distinction to the "schoolism" and materialist roots of the medical model. It is my sincere hope that in reading this book, psychotherapists will be empowered to provide their clients with healing that transcends symptom relief and goes beyond the mechanistic application of techniques. I believe that if we can help individuals heal, we will collectively work to heal the world.

Chapter Two

The History of the Study of Mind: From Philosophy to Science and Back to Philosophy

What is the current state of psychotherapy today? The brief answer is that it appears to be in flux, at least in some circles. There is no doubt that the dominant view still holds sway. It is taught in most programs in which therapists are trained. It is held by many influential mental health professionals. Perhaps most importantly therapists are required to operate within this view in order to access payments from insurance companies and managed care organizations. This dominant approach to mental health is referred to in much of the literature as the medical model.

Understanding where we are now and how we got here is a necessary first step in working toward changing the situation. A historical view helps us see clearly which concepts developed over time and came to be normalized. Once we understand how concepts came to be normalized, we can begin to question them. In order to understand how holistic therapy can correct for the deficits in the current model, I am presenting a very brief history of some of the important moments in the evolution of how mental health came to be practiced as it is today. We will see that from philosophy to science, from medicine (including psychiatry) to psychology, there has been a push to understand the human mind as an epiphenomenon of the brain or, more broadly, of neurochemical processes (there are some advocates of including the nerves in and around the heart and the vagus nerve as important to mental functioning). The problem is that understanding the mind to be reducible to the body has led us in a direction that is not working.

While forces have pushed a materialist agenda, there have been counterforces in medicine, in parapsychology, and more recently in post-materialist psychology. These movements offer us some clues as to how we might go about improving our understanding of mental suffering and mental well-being and may offer some markers as to how adopting a holistic view can correct for the current deficiencies.

From Philosophy to Science

The history of science is the history of the exploration and elevation of the physical world. As early philosophers contemplated life, they took for granted the natural world around them. They set their sights on that which was beyond the natural universe. For Plato, this meant the Ideal, or Forms. He considered Forms to be abstractions and thus knowable only by the mind. They are not knowable by sense experience and have a higher level of reality than those things that are the concrete particulars that are manifestations of Forms (Duignan 2018). He thought that our five senses distorted the fundamental nature of reality (he was quite ahead of his time). From Plato's vantage point, the physical world was seen as inferior to the Ideal or Forms (Bauer 2015).

It was Plato's student Aristotle who established that the physical world was worthy of close observation and increased understanding (Bauer 2015). This, Bauer observed, was "science." Bauer (2015) credited Aristotle with one of the fundamental building blocks of the scientific method: that it is important to understand how physical things change over time if one wants to truly understand the physical world.

For a very long period of time in Western civilization, the works of the Greek philosophers like Plato and Aristotle were the foundation of higher learning. Indeed, it was philosophers who rose to leadership in institutions of higher learning (Wootten 2015). This held sway until the Scientific Revolution.

Wootten (2015) argued that Western science was invented between 1572 and 1704 and continues to dominate human existence to this day. From the late sixteenth century until the early eighteenth century, there was a shift in European academic interest from philosophy to natural philosophy. Wootten argued that natural philosophy actually meant the natural sciences. What distinguished natural philosophy from philosophy was the test of experience.

But what is experience? In the scientific context, experience is comprised of those things that can be apprehended through the five traditional (embodied) senses, that is, our physically mediated interaction with the physical world. Wootten (2015) referred to the Scientific Revolution as new sense-perceptions. What made these perceptions possible was the invention of instruments to extend our human perceptions, such as the telescope and microscope. But what do we do with these experiences? How do we use them to make sense of our world?

In 1620, Francis Bacon, following Aristotle, asserted that inductive reasoning was the royal road to truth. He went even further. He developed a procedure to apply this form of reasoning. This procedure was to become the basis of the scientific method: hypothesis, experiment, conclusion. The word "experiment" has the same root as "experience" (Wootten 2015). So "experiment" means using the five senses (potentially extended by instruments) to observe the physical world. We posit a hypothesis, then observe, and draw a conclusion as to whether our hypothesis is confirmed.

This is where mathematics enters the history of science. Observing nature can give us a lot of information. But measuring things and seeing how these measurements change over time in specified circumstances can yield more knowledge about the physical world. Wootten (2015) pointed to the "mathematization of nature" as one of the key features of the Scientific Revolution.

What the sociologists of science tell us at this point is that there is something else going on here: the traditional authorities, along with the traditional basis for authority, were discredited by the new natural philosophy. Scientists were replacing philosophers as the arbiters of reality. As Wootten (2015) stated, "The scientific revolution was, first and foremost, a revolt by the mathematicians against the authority of the philosophers" (209). The mathematicians/scientists won because they had patronage. They had patronage because they could use their observations in ways that made people money: sailors could navigate the ocean more accurately; surveyors could measure land more accurately. The new way of looking at the world had clear economic advantages for some. And thus, science became the preferred method over philosophy to know about the world.

To be sure, observing yielded information. But perhaps more importantly, the scientific method could be used to predict: where do you need to mount the cannon to get the cannonball to hit the desired wall? The answers to such questions were believed to be based on the laws of nature. The great thinkers of the Scientific Revolution concluded that their observations would yield the immutable laws of nature. By the nineteenth century, a mathematician asserted that Newton's laws could predict anything that could happen in the future.

And here we have the basics of science: it is the investigation of the physical world with the five senses. These observations are "operationalized" or quantified in order to perform mathematical operations on them. The process unfolds as theory, observation/measurement/mathematical operation, conclusion. The purpose of this process may be pure knowledge, but it is highly desirable to be able to use the information to predict (or control).

This process has led to immense benefits for portions of the human population, certainly not everybody but many. It has been devastating for some other forms of life, indeed, for the health of the earth itself. But in the short term, those who had replaced the old authorities benefited greatly, as many humans did.

The optimism of nineteenth century scientists concerning the value of their growing corpus of knowledge perhaps reached its apogee in the early twentieth century. Warner (1995) has argued that by the first half of the nineteenth century, science had moved from a body of knowledge or a set of techniques to a value system—an ideology. This ideological shift perhaps peaked in the 1920s with the birth of the Vienna Circle and the Berlin Society for Empirical Philosophy.

These two groups of scientists, mathematicians, and philosophers were meeting to promote the "Scientific World-Conception" (Romizi 2012). The Vienna Circle and the Berlin Society for Empirical Philosophy were both working to promote logical positivism as more than the best way to understand the physical world. They stressed that it was the only proper epistemology with which to understand reality. In 1928, a subgroup of Vienna Circle members along with other political actors formed the Ernst Mach Society in order to popularize and publicize the Scientific World-Conception (Romizi 2012). That is, logical positivism was believed to be an appropriate basis for a comprehensive worldview.

The worldview advanced the notion that because only that which can be directly observed is real (Heineman 1981), only matter is real. This means that they dismissed any theoretical speculation as untrustworthy: any appeal to the metaphysical was meaningless. Only matter mattered. They thus promoted a strict materialist ontology. Romizi (2012) has noted that the Scientific World-Conception promoted "a particular value to science and a special epistemological status to scientific knowledge…scientific knowledge is the only 'real' knowledge" (213).

Romizi (2012) and Uibel (2022) have suggested that there was a distinct political agenda associated with the work of the Vienna Circle particularly. Romizi has asserted that this worldview was in stark opposition to the authority held by the Catholic Church and forces of Christianity, nationalism, and the national socialists. Logic and empiricism were believed to be the antidote to the emotional rhetoric of the fascists. One may have a great deal of sympathy for this political agenda. Yet even if our politics are aligned with the political implications of logical positivism, we must also recognize that their worldview blinkers much that gives human life depth and meaning.

One may not be surprised to learn of the antipathy of some members of the Vienna Circle with the growing knowledge being generated by quantum physicists. Bauer (2015) summarized quantum mechanics in these terms. The atom was supposed to be the smallest particle in the world, the thing upon which everything else was built. But lo, the atom had parts. And it got worse. Energy was understood to be a wave, that is, it should flow smoothly through space (and time). But predictions about how radioactive energy should act failed. The only explanation was that perhaps sometimes energy was comprised of tiny particles (called quanta), and these quanta did not move through space but seemed to disappear altogether and reappear somewhere else that was not predictable. One could forecast the chance of it showing up somewhere, but one can only know the probability of it doing so. This was termed the "quantum jump." Indeed, it appears that electrons regularly perform quantum leaps. Worse yet, on the subatomic level, one can't really measure particles. Any instrument sensitive enough to measure a subatomic particle will, in the process of measuring that particle, alter the trajectory of it. Known as the Heisenberg uncertainty principle, this finding means that one can't observe something without changing it. The act of observing affects that which we are observing. Suddenly our solid, predicable, observable world is not so solid, predictable, or knowable through observation. Ironically, the scientific method ultimately has raised questions about the ability of the scientific method to reveal everything important about existence. Science seemed to be casting suspicion upon scientism and the scientific method. Quantum mechanics, applied to biology and psychology or life in general, has undermined a mechanistic view of these processes (van Strien 2022). As van Strien (2022) has observed, "Quantum mechanics had shown that there was a fundamental limit to the scope of science, and quantum mechanics was often connected (not in the least by leading quantum physicists themselves) to speculative ideas about religion, free will, psychology, and organic life" (360).

The threat to the scientific worldview leveled by quantum mechanics was largely ignored by many scientists. Indeed, while quantum physics cast suspicion on the universality of the scientific method, the field of medicine was moving to bring itself into greater alignment with the scientists.

Medicine and Science

Psychotherapy is aimed at healing. Healing has been the domain of medicine since its inception. Warner (1995) has argued that the history of medicine and the history of science exist in a complicated relationship to each other. The Venn diagram of science and medicine, Warner (1995) suggested, has a significant common area around their "shared exploration of how natural knowledge is produced, organized, and deployed" (165).

Certainly, the practice of helping humans overcome physical dysfunction and disease predates the rise of natural philosophy. Early in human history, physical maladies were believed to have nonmaterial causes, including the effect of a spell or demonic possession (Rhodes et al 2022). Such nonphysical explanations continued to be used to account for the remediation of maladies (for example mesmerism, or magnetism). Bauer (2015) has suggested that the field of medicine changed around 1315. At that time, universities began to teach human anatomy based on observations made by means of human dissection. By 1543, Vesalius had exhorted anatomists to supplement the authority of ancient philosopher-physicians with the observations they made with their own eyes. As was the case with the development of science, medicine was moving from speculative theory to theory based on observation (Bauer 2015).

Between roughly 1500 and 1700, science came to mean this: you could only attend to that which could be apprehended with the five senses (or instruments that extend those senses). In other words, you could only ask questions about the physical world. The human body is physical. It makes sense on the face of it that the scientific method could help physicians learn about the human body. This knowledge could be used to help people experiencing a deviation in physical processes that leads to suffering.

Warner (1995) has been clear: part of the reason medicine was adopting a growing identity as scientifically grounded had socio-political ramifications. In seventeenth century London, when mathematicians and natural philosophers were gaining patronage for their financially beneficial discoveries (Wootten 2015), the impulse to identify a profession with empiricism brought a competitive edge to the medical marketplace (Warner 1995). By 1923, the term "biomedicine" appeared for the first time in Dorland's *Medical Dictionary*. It was defined there as "clinical medicine based on the principles of physiology and biochemistry" (Quirke, 2008).

Medicine, as a science, developed a standardized process to approach illness. Verhaeghe (2004) described the procedure as such: "The...patient displays a number of symptoms that are collated by the doctor so as to identify—diagnose—a distinct syndrome. This is done in accordance with an established knowledge that maintains both a notion of etiology and a clear diagnostic distinction between health and illness. In this way, the doctor makes a diagnosis, usually with the help of various instruments (thermometer, stethoscope, etc.), forms a prognosis, and suggests a treatment on the basis of her observations. The intent is to return to the status quo ante, the earlier state" (3).

This process, termed "the medical model," is the paradigmatic basis for mental health treatment today. As we will see shortly, the medical model, or biomedical model, has come to be the dominant orienting model for psychiatry. Nonetheless, there was an important pushback against this model. According to Alvarez, Pagani, and Meucci (2011), Roy Grinker coined the term "biopsychosocial model" in 1954. Engel adopted the term in arguing against the purely biomedical model. The biomedical model, he observed, is a "classic factor-analytic approach" (Engel 1980, 535) and thus is appropriate to the bench scientist but not the physician. He elaborated: While the bench scientist can with relative impunity single out and isolate for sequential study components of an organized whole, the physician does so at the risk of neglect of, if not injury to, the object of study, the patient" (536).

Engel (1980) called for the adoption of a systems model based on the work of Paul Weiss and Ludwig van Bertalanffy. He suggested that a more encompassing approach to patients' functioning would preserve the humanity of the patient and their attributes as a person. Engel was clear that in adopting a biopsychosocial model of patient care, one was not leaving the safety and comfort of science. Instead, he asserted that a systems model is a scientific model but renders the practice of medicine more "holistic and humanistic" (543).

In 1999, the World Health Organization added the word "spiritual" to the biopsychosocial model, arguing that spiritual issues are vital to health (Saad and de Medeiros 2020). "Psyche" is Greek for soul/spirit or personality or mind. Thus, a psychological approach *should* include considerations included by the term "spirituality." Yet mainstream psychiatry and psychology have to a large degree rejected such investigation and consigned such questions to the field of parapsychology. For many forms of holistic therapy spirituality is an important focus of treatment.

As much as the knowledge generated by hard sciences helped medicine, up until the 1960s, the practice of medicine was considered an art and was based on expert opinion, clinical experience, and clinical judgment (Sur and Dahm 2011). By the 1960s, physicians were importing biomedical sciences into their practice to enhance the "scientific basis for clinical care" (Sur and Dahm 2011, 487). These scientific discoveries that enhance the practice of medicine multiplied as time progressed. By 1990, Guyatt had declared a "Scientific Medicine." The following year Guyatt renamed his approach to medicine "Evidence-Based Medicine" (Sur and Dahm 2011).

Evidence-based medicine is premised on the application of medical interventions based on the published findings of research that can demonstrate the success of an intervention. As Holmes (2000) noted, "Evidence-Based Medicine argues that medical practice should model itself on scientific method and that all interactions with patients should be guided by the falsifiability principle: only those interventions which have been shown by rigorous tests to be effective should be implemented" (92).

The value of the research findings that physicians were to apply to their clinical work became an important consideration. In the '60s and '70s, Tom Chalmers stressed the importance of the Randomized Controlled Trial (RTC), and later the meta-analysis of RTCs, as the best kind of evidence to help physicians to decide how to treat their patient (Sur and Dahm 2011).

The randomized controlled trial and/or meta-analyses of RTCs are the gold standard of EBM. The RTC method is based on the quantification of objective, externally observable changes to bodies (matter) in controlled circumstances. Once the measures are collected, they are subject to statistical manipulation. In other words, however much the worldview of the Vienna Circle may be challenged today, whatever one may think about the challenges that quantum mechanics may pose to the normative view of science imposed by the logical positivists, the research upon which evidence-based medicine is premised is logical positivist through and through. This is the world of the medical specialization of psychiatry.

As Sur and Dahm (2011) noted, although evidence-based medicine is taught in several prominent medical schools, there is significant criticism of this approach. Most notably, the application of aggregated data to an individual may deprive the individual of optimal care. Perhaps the most significant objection to EBM is the potential for abuse on the part of health care policymakers and third-party payers, justified on the basis of best available evidence rather than on the need of an individual patient (Sur and Dahm 2011).

I must stress here that the issue is not whether the scientific method can illuminate important information about the functioning of the human body and the amelioration of physical maladies. The question is if this is the only legitimate way to acquire useful information about human functioning and especially about human mental functioning. "Illness" is not the same as "disease." Ventriglio, Torales, and Bughra (2017) differentiated disease and illness in this way: "Disease literally as dis-ease, meaning that it deals with pathology, which is what doctors are trained to identify and manage. On the other hand, illness is what patients are interested in, as the impact of disease occurs on their functioning, relationships and social interactions" (3).

It is worth stressing here that the difficulty in resolving mind-body dualism is not in recognizing that mind and body are aspects of a single phenomenon but in falling into material monism, where mind is believed only to be an epiphenomenon of body. The resolution of dualism was to erase the fundamental reality of mind.

As we review the rise of science and materialism, we must keep in mind that if there is any aspect of human functioning that is not reducible to material processes, if mind is not an epiphenomenon of brain, then the scientific method and evidence-based medicine, the medical model of psychological functioning, and the value of evidence-based practices for psychotherapy cannot give us a complete understanding of mental suffering or well-being.

Psychology and Psychotherapy

The first piece of business to address when thinking about a history of psychology is to delimit what we mean by psychology. In the standard conceptualization of psychology by psychologists, we see a breakdown of the term into "psyche," which means "mind" or "soul," and "ology," which means "the study of something." But as we have seen, the study of something came to mean the scientific, materialist, quantified, objectivist study of something. Thus when one reviews the history of psychology, one finds the history of the Western scientific study of the mind. As Wilber (2000) noted, people had been engaged in the empirical (meaning knowing through observation and experience) study of mind for millennia. Particularly in the East, the mind/spirit had been the object of introspective and contemplative practices. We will look at this at more length in the chapter on integral philosophy and psychology.

In the Western scientific tradition, there are two important groups of writers, thinkers, and researchers that have contributed to psychotherapy: psychology and psychoanalysis. Both were conceived by medical doctors. We will look first at psychology.

Western Psychology

Western thought is typically traced back to the Greek culture. In ancient Greece, scholars were philosophers. Psychology began as a subset of philosophy. As the sciences go, psychology remained in philosophy departments of institutions of higher learning until relatively late.

The Greek philosophers understood what we now conceptualize as mental illness—like physical illnesses—to be the work of demons or gods (Hunt 2007). Hippocrates (460–377 BCE) was among the first to posit that mental illness was, in fact, a dysfunction of the brain. But this notion was abandoned as philosophers considered the relationship between mind and body.

One philosopher of note in the ensuing debate is Plato. He argued that what is real is the Ideal: that which exists as an abstraction. He believed that perception with the five senses is unreliable, as it distorts the Ideal. Instead, reflection and reason were the appropriate epistemological tools to know what is real and fundamental. This placed metaphysics at the core of psychology. As psychology moved from philosophy to science, this view was turned on its head.

Somewhat before the Vienna Circle declared that the only legitimate object of study was matter and that the only legitimate method of study was the logical manipulation of objective measurements, there had been a growing zeitgeist toward scientism, which is reflected in the history of Western psychology. The year 1879 is often cited as the birth of the field of psychology. Certainly, it is the year psychology moved from philosophy to science. For in that year, William Wundt set up the first laboratory at the University of Leipzig. There is some disagreement about Wundt's work (Asthana 2015). Hunt (2007), for example, has stressed that Wundt's first research project was to measure the time lag between stimulus and perception. Given that Wundt was a medical doctor and a lecturer in physiology, some writers stress that his early work was on physiological psychology (Hunt 2007). Yet Asthana (2015) has argued that Wundt has been misinterpreted and misunderstood. Asthana stressed that Wundt replaced the word psyche with the word *geist* (even though the words mean roughly the same thing) in order to stress that he was interested in mind, not soul. Wundt understood mind to be experience and not to be circumscribed by physical reductionism, according to Asthana. Wundt understood the principal method of study for the mind to be introspection, or the observation of "inner private mental processes as a form of scientific data" (Asthana 2015, 245).

William James, often cited as the father of American psychology, rose to prominence shortly after Wundt. In 1875, James taught the first psychology class in the United States at Harvard University. His appointment at Harvard was to teach anatomy and physiology. Over time, he moved to psychology, then philosophy. As the "scientization" of psychology moved it out of the realm of philosophy, James appears to have had some ambivalence about the move. Like Wundt, he was a physician who taught anatomy and physiology. He was clear in his writing that psychology was in line to become a natural science, even though it was not there yet (Campbell 2017). And yet, as James turned from medicine to psychology and then to philosophy, he embraced metaphysics. It would seem that he could not finally fully accept the materialist project of science as the best way of fully understanding the mind.

In spite of the efforts of James and Wundt, most historians of psychology agree that behaviorism soon became the dominant school of psychology in the West (Asthana 2015). With the rise of behaviorism, subjectivity was abandoned as a legitimate arena of study in psychology, and the positivist agenda became firmly fixed.

This situation has begun to change to a small degree. We see now the rise of post-materialist psychology. A small number of psychologists who study consciousness and spirituality have suggested that materialism can no longer hold as the dominant ontology if one wishes to understand the human mind.

Parapsychology

During the years that science and the scientific study of the mind or psychology were becoming routinized, there was another group of people who were also interested in the mind. These were those who studied esotericism, the occult, and psychic phenomena, otherwise known as magic. According to Hutton (2019), there was a revival of ritual magic in Great Britain around 1867. One of the leading figures in the occult revival was Eliphas Zahed Levi. Levi and other occultists embarked on a mission to realize the potential of the human mind by tapping into imagination and willpower as well as by accessing altered states of consciousness. The practice of magic was seen as a form of therapy to develop the divine within the individual. It seemed clear to some that the occult and psychology were equally concerned about the nature and potential of the mind.

This revival was heralded by the Rosicrucian Society. The Rosicrucians identified as Christians who studied cabala, hermetic texts, and included Enochian magic in their rituals (Hutton 2019). Of interest here is the fact that an early Rosicrucian defined magic as a "psychological branch of science, dealing with sympathetic effects of stones, drugs, and living substances upon the imaginative and reflective ca-pacities" (King 1970, quoted in Hutton 2019, 75). We see here that magic and the occult are viewed as psychological phenomena. In other words, psychological phenomena can also encompass experiences that are not mediated by the five senses. Psychological phenomena include experiences of the imagination and other forms of subjectivity, includ-ing reflection. This pulls the idea of psychology out of the world of Western science.

The period that saw the creation of scientific psychology also saw a rise in spiritualism. Spiritualism is the belief in the persistence of some aspect of one's personality or mind beyond death. The system of thought is not as psychologically focused as the Rosicrucian system of high magic, but it is noteworthy that at the time of the rise of ma-terialist psychology there was a popular movement that purported to demonstrate that some aspect of mind exists beyond the viability of the body. The popularity of the belief may be reflected in some statis-tics. For example, one of the spiritualist groups in Britain was estimat-ed to have about twenty-five thousand members before the First World War. In Britain, one estimate is that spiritualism peaked in the 1930s at around two thousand spiritualist societies (Bruce 2020).

In spite of the fact that the spiritualists believed that the soul could live past the life of the body, they were nonetheless committed to the scientific study of occult phenomena. According to the American So-ciety for Psychical Research website, in 1885, a group of spiritualists, along with none other than William James and several other noted intellectuals, founded the organization. The American Society was fashioned after its British precursor, the Society for Psychical Research (SPR), founded in 1882 (Eaton 2022). The SPR was founded by spir-itualists to investigate thought transference (telepathy), mesmerism (the power of hypnotic suggestion), mediumship, Odic force (an en-ergy or life force believed to operate on physical entities), and appari-tions and haunted houses (University of Cambridge n.d.). It must be noted that the societies were dedicated to the newly growing scientific zeitgeist: their aim was to use scientific methods to explore the possibility that soul or spirit existed beyond death and hence potentially independently of the body. In the words of Eaton (2022), members of the two societies "wanted to prove beyond a shadow of a doubt, and perhaps more importantly to persuade others, that there was indeed a supernatural world beyond the senses" (112). In other words, the strict materialism was questioned by some members of the nascent community of psychologists.

Also in 1875, the Theosophical Society was created by Helena Blavatsky and Henry Steele Olcott. The Theosophical Society was dedicated to the study of the "hidden mysteries of Nature" (Hutton 2019). Blavatsky was highly influenced by Eastern traditions, to the degree that she subordinated Western esoteric traditions to those of India. She claimed to have a psychic link to the Mahatmas, semi-divine beings of a clearly Eastern bent. Blavatsky's psychic abilities were later determined to be spurious by the Society for Psychical Research in 1884 (Hutton 2019). Of interest here is the degree to which, through the Theosophical Society, Westerners were being introduced to Eastern thought, and there were nascent attempts to reconcile the two.

Today, we see that the possible connection between occult phenomena and psychology continues in the field of parapsychology (beside psychology). The ASPR currently focuses on the nature of consciousness. The researchers at the Rhine Research Center (originally housed at Duke University) define parapsychology as "the broader study of consciousness and the mind (Rhine n.d.). Parapsychological researchers continue to explore the nature of mind and consciousness, even though their work is not accepted in mainstream psychology. And that is the point of this excursus. If a holistic approach to helping the mind is to reject the bio-reductionist view of mind, it may be that reviewing the work of those who have studied the mind from a nonmaterialist perspective and those who have studied the potentials of mind that challenge the boundaries of mainstream psychology may provide us with valuable insights and tools.

Psychoanalysis

That Freud was a materialist is hardly debated among psychoanalysts and other scholars. Freud began his work as so many early figures in psychology did, as a medical doctor: a neurologist. As a physician, he specialized in the diagnosis and treatment of brain damage and disease (Hunt 2007). He firmly believed that there was a neurological explanation for mental suffering (Barford, Geerardyn, and van der Gertusvan 2002). Although, as Barford, Geerardyn and van der Vijver (2002) contend, psychology-oriented commentators on Freudian work have asserted that he ultimately left behind his bio-reductionist aspirations.

Perhaps saying that Freud abandoned his materialist views is misleading. There is no doubt that at some point after the publication of *Project for a Scientific Psychology*, Freud stopped trying to formulate a biological theory of mental suffering (Hunt 2007). This may be due more to the shift in the focus of his work than any shift in ontology. Freud turned away from an attempt to explain his patients' experiences in terms of neurological activity and tried instead to understand how the human mind works based on his case studies. He turned to listening and attempted to understand the inner experiences of his patients. This is not in keeping with the then-dominant view of what constitutes good science. It may be in part due to this seemingly non-scientific approach to the mind that Freud is not covered in detail in most academic psychology programs today.

Among many of the mental processes that interested Freud, perhaps the most controversial was his interest in thought transference, or telepathy. He clearly feared that if he pursued his interest, psychoanalysis might suffer as a legitimate form of treatment. Nonetheless, he came to be convinced that this phenomenon was a regular occurrence in analysis. The idea of telepathy in analysis has never successfully been suppressed. Today, we see the concept being openly discussed among analysts as unconscious communication that occurs in the analytic field (see, for example, volume 39, no. 4–5 of *Psychoanalytic Inquiry* for a collection of articles on the topic). Again, the point is this: a holistic approach to therapy may benefit from gathering and using information about the client that comes to the therapist from communication that is not verbal or paralinguistic. Indeed, clinical intuition (see Stickle and Arnd-Caddigan 2019 and Arnd-Caddigan 2021) may be a central feature of holistic psychotherapy.

Psychotherapy, the Medical Model, and Evidence-Based Practice

Hunt (2007) has noted that Wundt, one of the originators of the young science of psychology, was dismayed by the number of his students who used their knowledge to provide psychotherapy. Hunt referred to the practice as "applied science." Yet there are many disciplines that did not necessarily define themselves as applied scientists who also came to provide psychotherapeutic services. Among these are clinical social workers, marriage and family therapists, and pastoral counselors. They were brought into line fairly quickly.

In 1953, Hans Eysenck, a psychologist, declared that psychotherapy was ineffective (Lebow and Jenkins 2018). Eysenck decided on variables that he thought should constitute effectiveness and measured people who had received therapy and those who did not in terms of his identified outcomes. He found that people who did not receive treatment showed improvement and thus determined that therapy had no value. This spurred the push for psychotherapy research (Lebow and Jenkins 2018) and may have been the first impulse toward what today is called "evidence-based practice" in psychotherapy.

Of course, we have to specify exactly what it works for. As noted above, the medical discipline had created a template for how it went about its practice. A physician observes objective symptoms, which, when presented in combinations, determine a diagnosis. The diagnosis is then treated with methods known to be effective to eliminate the cause of the disease or, failing the ability to do so, at minimum ameliorate the distressing symptoms. This model was adopted in psychiatry for the identification of mental illnesses.

In 1952, the American Psychiatric Association published the *Diagnostic and Statistical Manual of Mental Disorders* (DSM) (Psychiatry. org, n.d.). This volume represented the official classification listing the symptom clusters for diagnoses of mental illnesses. The DSM is currently in its fifth edition and its eighth iteration (the third, fourth, and fifth editions all have revised versions). And yet there is still widespread disagreement over the classification system: "Increasing dissatisfaction with the validity of the criteria has become apparent with complaints that the criteria do not sufficiently differentiate disorders leading to high rates of diagnostic comorbidity, diagnoses lack specificity for selection of treatment, genetics fail to distinguish psychiatric disorders, and many observed syndromes do not fit any diagnostic definition" (Suris, Holliday, and North 2016, 1).

Much of the problem with the validity of the diagnoses that form the basis for current mental health treatment may be attributable to the fact that the categories were constructed on a completely subjective basis. They were determined by means of a vote, which was based on the experiences of those voting. Perhaps even more dauting, there is currently no objective biological test to determine if an individual has one of the diagnoses in the *DSM* (Thompson 2019). After decades of insisting that mental illnesses are biological, there remains no biological determinates for a diagnosis. And despite the claims made on popular websites, there is no clearly identifiable biological cause for most of the diagnoses in the *DSM* (Thompson 2019). As the popular saying goes, "correlation is not causation." The body and the mind are correlated, to be sure. The causal pathway is an ontological assumption.

If the diagnostic criteria are not valid, the notion that therapy should be targeted toward these labels falls. And yet this is exactly the direction evidence-based practice in psychotherapy (EBP) has gone. The logic of EBP is that once there are specific symptoms and specific diagnoses that are the correct target for psychotherapy, determining whether or not a form of therapy is effective is simply a matter of measuring symptoms before and after treatment. In step with physicians who adopted evidence-based medicine, psychotherapists were told that they must only use what has been empirically demonstrated to work. To accomplish this, treatment must be standardized in order to ensure that all research subjects are getting the same thing. Thus, the treatment is manualized, and those who deliver the treatment for research purposes must be able to demonstrate adherence to the treatment manual. Likewise, the subjects must be similar to ensure that one is delivering treatment to people with the same disease. For this reason, subjects must have a single diagnosis (no comorbidities), and usually they have a mild to moderate presentation of the diagnosis. These subjects are unlike the clients therapists typically work with. As is the case with evidence-based medicine, there is a hierarchy of forms of research that is used to determine the status of a form of treatment. But the recognition that the diagnostic categories that are being measured are themselves invalid plus the fact that the research subjects bear little resemblance to real life clients throws off the whole endeavor. Thus the results of the outcome studies that are supposed to guide our treatment are not applicable to our clients.

Thomas Insel, a psychiatrist and former head of the NIMH, is firmly committed to the medical model. Yet he unequivocally stated, "Simply put, mental illnesses are different from other illnesses. Our current approach is a disaster on many fronts. Not only is mental health care delivered ineffectively, but it is mostly accessed during a crisis and strategically focused only on relieving symptoms and not on helping people recover" (Insel 2022, xix).

A point that will become relevant as we move to models of holistic therapy is this: it is the logic of evidence-based practice that underlies a prohibition against integrating theoretical approaches and techniques to therapy. No integrated approach has the evidentiary status of a single theoretical approach. And how could it? In many cases, therapists make an in-session decision about what their client needs. They do not rely on formalized manuals to respond to their clients but on their deep connection to their client and a solid understanding of the client's intrapsychic and interpersonal dynamics (Stickle and Arnd-Caddigan 2019).

The current state of the medical model and evidence-based practice in mental health is this: the mental illnesses for which treatment should be targeted lack validity and often are not the actual focus of treatment. The methodology to gauge the effectiveness of a form of treatment renders the results inapplicable to actual clinical situations. We see that third-party payers have reduced the focus of treatment and the treatment options available to clients and providers. Many therapists have determined that the best way to provide what their clients need is to refuse to accept third-party payments, but this limits the people for whom comprehensive treatment is available.

And yet there has been dissent. The evidence-based practice model is based on highly manualized forms of treatment that represent different schools or theories or brands of psychotherapy. For example, there is Cognitive-Behavioral Therapy and Psychodynamic Psychotherapy and so forth. In fact, there are now at least five hundred different types of psychotherapy available today (Lilienfeld and Arkowitz 2012). The logic is that the techniques that are derived from and unique to a specific theoretical approach are the mutative factors in psychotherapy. However, there is a growing body of research that suggests that it is not the type of therapy that is important in mental healing. The researchers who study common factors agree that the type of therapy one uses does influence outcome, but it is not the major driver of client change. Indeed, it has been found repeatedly that most forms of therapy have roughly equivalent outcomes and that there are a number of factors that are common to many of the approaches to treatment that lead to client change (Wampold 2010). There are a number of therapists who feel comfortable integrating different approaches to treatment on the basis of this common factors research (Stricker 2001).

Back to Philosophy of Mind: Full Circle

Previously, I have discussed cosmopsychism as a possible worldview that addresses mind qua mind and not just body (Arnd-Caddigan 2021). Keppler and Shani (2020) have referred to cosmopsychism as a holistic form of panpsychism. There are many forms of panpsychism (Arnd-Caddigan 2021). The most basic feature of this position is the view that "there is only one kind of thing but it features physical and mental properties" (Bruntrip 2017, 51, quoted in Arnd-Caddigan 2021, 15). In other words, like dualistic views of reality, there is an acknowledgment that mind and matter are both real. Contrary to dualism, panpsychism holds that they are both aspects of a single unitary universe.

In this worldview, matter is defined as that which has physical properties: it exists in time and space, it has volume and mass, etc. Matter is objective; we can apprehend it with our five senses (or extensions of those senses through technology), and when several people look at an object, there is some agreement about what they perceive. Mind, on the other hand, is subjective (and intersubjective). It does not occupy space. It is *qualia*, or the experience of what it's like. Mind is often referred to as "consciousness" in much of the literature.

There are several reasons why it is difficult to assert that mind is a side effect of activity in the brain: first, there are living organisms on earth that do not have brains yet demonstrate "forms of perception and behavioral plasticity, information processing, anticipation, memory, learning, valence, problem-solving, communication, and cooperation" (Keppler and Shani 2020, 2). In addition, Brabant (2016) noted that the fact that mind can influence the body is indicative of the fact that mind cannot be created by the body: the effect does not influence the cause. He noted that the most obvious example of this is the placebo and nocebo effects as well as observations that meditation (an altered state of consciousness) changes the brain. Brabant (2016) also noted that there appears to be enhanced subjective experience in instances when brain activity is reduced or even completely absent.

He noted experiments with psychedelics and near-death experiences (NDEs) as examples. We would expect that if the brain caused experience, there would be more brain activity when there was heightened experience, not less. In the case of NDEs, it would appear that subjective experience and memory can continue with no discernible brain activity. Egnor (2018) is a neurologist who has worked with a number of patients who are severely neurologically compromised: they have extensive damage to their brains. He has observed, at first to his surprise, that in the face of profoundly deficient brain structures, individuals are able to demonstrate full mental functioning.

The evidence Egnor (2018) cites is based to a large degree on the research of Roger Sperry. The latter studied persons who had had their corpus colosseum severed: the right hemisphere and left hemisphere of their brains were not in communication with each other. Over and over, while some physical anomalies were found in these patients, their minds—including their sense of agency—remained intact. Egnor (2018) also cited the work of Wilder Pennfield, who induced seizures in patients by stimulating the brain. While Pennfield could induce a physical seizure, he could not produce an intellectual seizure; mental functioning remained intact. Egnor's (2018) conclusion is that there is part of every human being that is not reducible to their brain. He chooses to refer to this aspect of humanity as a soul. Philosophers of mind tend to choose to refer to this as "mind" or "consciousness." The point is that there is an aspect of humans that is not material: there is something more.

In the same vein, Baruss and Mossbridge (2017) discussed terminal lucidity. This is when a person with a diagnosed cognitive impairment (like dementia) suddenly has a brief return of mental clarity. Autopsies confirm sufficient brain pathology to lead one to believe that mental clarity is not due to the brain being restored. Baruss and Mossbridge (2017) also cited findings that strongly suggest that consciousness survives beyond death. In the research, mediums—people who appear to be able to "communicate with invisible intelligence [discarnates] or receive 'energy' from other dimensions of reality" (90)—must be able to supply information that could not have been known by other means. Finally, Brabant noted savant syndrome as an indication that knowledge can be more than the result of combining or reorganizing existing knowledge. He gave several examples of creation and problem-solving that appear to originate outside of the individual's store of knowledge. All of these areas of research suggest that mind can exist independently of the brain.

And then there is what has come to be widely known among philosophers of mind as the "hard problem." In 1995 philosopher David Chalmers coined the term and observed that in distinction to the hard problem, "The easy problems of consciousness are those that seem directly susceptible to the standard methods of cognitive science, whereby a phenomenon is explained in terms of computational or neural mechanisms" (2). Cognitive scientists can investigate the neural mechanisms that are active when one carries out specific functions. But cognitive science cannot explain why certain organisms are the subjects of experience. His conclusion was that experience—or mind, or consciousness, or *qualia*—is fundamental: it is not reducible to physical operations. In the materialist explanation there is always a magic black box moment in which something physical turns into something with no physical properties. Rather than rely on magic, Chalmers preferred to suggest that the only explanation is that mind is fundamental; it is not reducible to any physical activity: it exists in the universe as part of the universe. Mind and matter are "not viewed as two interacting substances, but as correlated projections from a common ground" (Brabant 2016, 350).

We see here repeated reasons why mind is not reducible to brain. This idea has been embraced by a growing number of scholars from various disciplines. While the forms of panpsychism all recognize that mind is fundamental, there is some disagreement concerning the question as to whether mind is always coincident with physical matter or if mind can exist apart from physical matter. The question also goes the other way: are there physical things that do not experience? I, of course, don't know. My intuition is that while a tree might experience,

I don't think a chair does. I think there are physical things that don't experience. Therefore, it seems to me that the inverse might be true: there are experiences that exist outside of physicality.

Of all of the competing forms of panpsychism that exist, cosmopsychism seems to be getting the lion's share of attention among post-materialist scholars and practitioners. Before I address cosmopsychism, let me discuss both dualism and panpsychism. Dualism is the view that mind and brain exist as separate realities. Michael Egnor (2018) wrote a tight popular-level article discussing his embrace of dualism. Dualism posits that mind and matter are two different realities. Panpsychists, on the other hand, see mind and matter as two aspects of a singular underlying reality. In some forms of panpsychism, mind and matter always coexist, so that an atom has a mind or perhaps a protomind. Cosmopsychists tend to endorse the idea that the universe has an external manifestation, which is matter, and an internal manifestation, which is mind. Mind is the "cosmic level of consciousness serving as the ultimate bedrock of experiential reality" (Keppler and Shani 2020, 3). In other words, all individual instances of mind—your mind, my mind, perhaps the mind of the tree—are instances or aspects of the singular all-pervasive Mind. As instances of the singular Mind, all individual instantiations are ontologically connected, just like the individual mushrooms you see in your yard are actually connected through a single mycelium underground.

Furthermore, the form of cosmopsychism on which I base my version of a mind-centered psychotherapy is understood to be participatory. That is, in a bi-directional manner, all individual minds affect each other and the universal mind, and the universal mind affects all individual instantiations of it. This extends to the therapy: the therapist and client affect each other in a reciprocal, mutually influential relationship. This is what Relational analysts have called a "two-person psychology" (Aron 1990).

The implications of this for mental well-being and holistic psychotherapy are profound. To be holistic, one must be able to perceive the individual and the mental connection between the individual and all other individuals as well as the cosmic ground of mindedness. Holistic therapy can offer us an antidote to the current "cerebro-centric" approach to clients. This means that the therapist must be ever mindful of how they are affecting the client's current presentation as well as how the client is affecting the therapist's subjective experience.

Conclusion

Today, the dominant approach to psychotherapy is the medical model. Psychotherapists who bill third parties (like Medicaid or private insurance companies) must deliver the type of therapy the entity dictates. Psychotherapists who bill a third party must demonstrate that their work is medically necessary, meaning the work is aimed at the reduction of symptoms of a mental health diagnosis, even if the diagnoses available demonstrate limited validity and reliability.

Moreover, the amelioration of symptoms is not the goal of some forms of psychotherapy. For example, Psychodynamic psychotherapy is aimed at client self-awareness and the loosening of rigid unconscious patterns. Client-centered Therapy is targeted to help clients achieve self-actualization. Many therapists work to help their clients achieve a sense of well-being. There are many ways therapy can help a person, and the resolution of symptoms of a diagnosis is often seen as a proximal objective but not the ultimate goal.

We have seen that this situation is the result of the medicalization of therapy, and the scientization of medicine. Science, as noted, came into being to learn about the material world. It shifted over time from a method to learn about the world to the notion that the material world was the only aspect of reality that was worthy of study, and it shifted again to the notion that the material world is the whole of reality. But if psychotherapy deals with the mind and the mind is not material, then the entire edifice crumbles.

We have also seen in the history of psychology and psychoanalysis some dissent to the notion that the mind is purely material. A holistic approach to psychotherapy may represent an alternative to the medical model. In constructing this alternative it may benefit us to go back to our roots and learn from people who have explored the mind from a nonmaterialist perspective.

Holistic Practice Points

- If holistic psychotherapy is to be an alternative to the medical model, it must move beyond bio-reductionism and transcend the narrow focus on diagnostic categories and symptom reduction. This means that we address the causes, processes, expressions, and effects of mental suffering in all of its manifestations that our clients experience.
- A post-materialist worldview suggests that mind is not brain. Furthermore, cosmopsychism suggests that minds are all instantiations of a universal mind. This is the basis for the understanding that individuals' minds are connected.

Chapter Three

Elements of Holistic Approaches

We saw in the last chapter that the medical model is not particularly well-suited for the treatment of mental suffering. A better approach may be holistic. But what exactly is a holistic form of psychotherapy? If you do an Internet search of the term, you'll come up with not only a dizzying number of websites, but you will also see that what is practiced as holistic therapy varies a great deal. The academic literature uses the term "biopsychosocial" to address more holistic approaches to therapy. Popular literature has embraced the term "holistic," with the understanding that at minimum, such an approach includes biological, psychological, social, and often spiritual considerations of human functioning.

In this chapter, we will look at various ways holistic therapy has been conceptualized. One mainstream therapy website called Verywell Mind suggests that any therapy that combines traditional and nontraditional approaches to well-being qualifies as a holistic therapy (Verywellmind.com, n.d.). The website lists four categories of holistic therapy: eclectic/integrative therapy, mind-body therapy, somatic therapy, and spiritual therapy. I have used these categories as a heuristic to look at several approaches to conceptualizing this construct. Specific modalities under these headings include bio-reductionist approaches that treat mental suffering by physical manipulation. These approaches are justified based on the theory that mind is the result of the activity of the autonomic nervous system. Other approaches emphasize the importance of addressing spiritual aspects of psyche to foster well-being. Yet other approaches advocate using a wide variety of theoretical perspectives and techniques in an effort to help clients heal by engaging mind, body, spirit, and social/cultural issues and an understanding of the role of energy in healing.

Thompson (2019, 2020, 64-71) is a social worker, and as such, it may not be surprising that he stresses the need to include social considerations in a holistic approach to mental well-being. He uses the work of sociologists who fall under the category of symbolic interactionists, or interactionists, as well as existential philosophers. He has also emphasized the need to return our focus to emotions; he has pointed out that clients do not come in complaining of thoughts but rather of feelings.

Somatic Therapies

If we conceptualize the mind as an epiphenomenon or side effect of neurochemical processes, the mind and body can be reduced to body. From this perspective, any biological approach to mental well-being is holistic in that it includes considerations of both mind and body as a unit. This is the underlying premise of the somatic approaches to psychotherapy. Somatic Experiencing Therapy, Hakomi, and Sensorimotor Therapy are all examples of somatic therapies aimed at reducing mental suffering. They all teach that intervening at the site of the body is key to helping resolve emotional difficulties.

In the case of Somatic Experiencing Therapy, the underlying theory of effectiveness is based on Polyvagal theory. While many mind-body therapies acknowledge that one's mental state can influence their physical state, polyvagal theory takes the opposite tack: physiological activities create feelings. Porges (2022), the originator of polyvagal theory (which is the theoretical foundation of Somatic Experiencing

Therapy) has stated: "The need to feel safe is functionally our body speaking through our autonomic nervous system—influencing our mental and physical health, social relationships, cognitive processes, behavioral repertoire, and serving as a neurophysiological substrate upon which societal institutions dependent on cooperation and trust function are based (2022, 2).

The importance of this statement cannot be overstated. Porges (2022) attributes thought, feeling, behavior, and social institutions to human biology. Lest you think that the feeling of safety—an experience or mental phenomenon—is the first cause, Porges (2022) is clear: "Feelings of safety are operationally the product of cues of safety, via neuroception…downregulating autonomic states that support threat reactions and upregulating autonomic states that support interpersonal accessibility and homeostatic functions" (2). That is, a cue (i.e., an external, objectively observable, potentially measurable event) triggers a biological reaction that creates the subjective experience as well as interpersonal behavior.

The therapy itself is a form of treatment aimed at releasing what is believed to be a build-up of traumatic energy in the body. By engaging in physical actions that are believed to release this energy, the patient is cured of the symptoms of Post Traumatic Stress Disorder (LynLake Centers for Well-being n.d.)

Sensorimotor Therapy is another somatic approach to the treatment of mental suffering. The system places a great deal of emphasis on our organicity (Sensorimotor Psychotherapy Institute n.d.). I read this as an assertion that we are primarily material/bodies. There is an acknowledgment that there is a primary connectedness within the universe. The system also recognizes that "Mind, body and spirit are intimately related, essential aspects of each of us. We keep the whole person in mind and consider mind, body, and spirit in context and relationship, rather than work with these elements in isolation" (Sensorimotor Psychotherapy Institute n.d.). In spite of this apparent inclusivity, the focus of treatment is on "the body's movement, posture, and sensations" (Sensorimotor Psychotherapy Institute n.d.). Sensorimotor Therapy was founded by the cofounder of Hakomi.

While Hakomi is often discussed as a somatic therapy, its originator also refers to the system as a mind-body therapy. Indeed, Kurtz, who created Hakomi, endorsed a clearly post-materialist ontology. He stated that Hakomi is "about the nature of living beings and their differences from the material, mechanical realm…about the reality of consciousness and its place in therapy" (Kurtz 1990, 2). The Hakomi website states as a primary principle the fact that an individual is a unity composed of many parts, including the physical/metabolic, intrapsychic, interpersonal, family, cultural, and spiritual (Hakomi Institute, n.d.). This view is, I believe, the heart of holistic therapy. Nonetheless, we once again see in Hakomi a focus on the neurological system. Indeed, Kurtz's (1990) book is entitled *Body-Centered Psychotherapy*. The Hakomi practitioner guides the client's attention to physical sensations and, in some cases, uses a hands-on approach, touching the client to support or bring awareness to embodied reactions.

We see then in the forms of somatic therapy described a fundamental assumption that the body is the preferable site of interventions for some forms of mental suffering. We live in a culture in which we are taught that we are our bodies, and that mental suffering is a disease of the brain. If we are to help people identify as being more than a body (truly holistic), we must emphasize balance by giving prominence to the mind-spirit-social-energetic aspects of our being.

This point is important: psychotherapy is treatment of the psyche and thus aimed at reducing mental (which includes emotional) suffering. Thus, we must think through the implications of using interventions aimed at changing the body as a means to treat mental suffering. Holism requires that we understand that because a person is a singular whole, mental suffering implicates all of the aspects of a person, including their bodies. But it must, in my opinion, move beyond a bio-reductionist view of a person's suffering. Holistic therapy suggests that while techniques that focus on the body can be an important part of a holistic approach, somatic therapy in and of itself is not holistic because holistic treatment holds that mind, spirit, and connectedness are not biologically based phenomena and must be given equal attention in therapy.

There is an additional point in relation to somatic therapies. Our experiences of our bodies are, by definition, *qualia*. That is, they are mental. Our minds always mediate our experiences of our bodies. Furthermore, our ability to train our awareness on most mental activity requires a relatively well-developed capacity for abstraction: our ability to reflect on something that does not have a physical existence. For clients who are more concrete, it may be easier to help them toward reflecting on abstract mental contents and processes by first reflecting on the experience of something concrete. This means their bodies. By helping our clients reflect on somatic experiences, we are training them to reflect on mind. From this perspective, somatic therapies are powerful and often a first step in a holistic therapy but are not sufficient to constitute a holistic therapy in which mind is a central aspect.

Spiritual Therapy

While psyche means both mind and spirit, both William Wundt, one of the originators of Western psychology, and Sigmund Freud, the father of psychoanalysis, drew clear demarcations between their work and spirituality. As Dein (2010) remarked, "Throughout most of the twentieth century taking patients' religious beliefs and experiences seriously was generally considered taboo" (2010, 525). Yet William James and Carl Jung were both extremely interested in spirituality and its role in human mental functioning.

In James's (1958) watershed series of lectures, collected into the book *The Varieties of Religious Experiences*, he was unequivocal about the appropriateness for the nascent field of psychology to explore religious experiences: "the religious propensities of man must be at least as interesting as any other of the facts pertaining to his mental constitution. It would seem, therefore, that, as a psychologist, the natural thing for me would be to invite you to a descriptive survey of those religious propensities" (22). In other words, humans have religious and/or spiritual experiences. James argued we have a propensity to have such experiences. These subjective experiences are psychological and must be understood in order to understand human psychology.

Carl Jung was a student of Freud's. Religion and spirituality are central to Jungian analytical psychology as it was to Jung himself (Main 2006), so much so, in fact, that critics have accused Jung and Jungians of attempting to turn psychology into a religion. In discussing religion, Jung's focus was on personal experience over and above the trappings of organized religion. He believed that the psyche is fundamentally religious and that humans require religion in some form for mental well-being (Main 2006).

In spite of the influence of these early figures in psychology, as Dein (2010) noted, spirituality constituted the third rail in psychotherapy for a good bit of the history of the practice. Yet in the latter part of the twentieth century, psychology entered a post-positivist era, and both Positive Psychology and Transpersonal Psychology have brought spirituality back into focus (Pargament and Saunders 2007). Pargament and Saunders made two important points concerning the role of spirituality in mental functioning. First, spirituality can be a psychological resource: "specific spiritual beliefs and practices have been tied to improvements in health and well-being,... studies suggest that spirituality may offer a distinctive way of understanding and dealing with life's most disturbing problems" (Pargament and Saunders 2007, 3).

Their second point is that clinicians must be aware of the ways that spirituality can cause or exacerbate mental suffering. They concluded that "the emerging literature in the psychology of religion and spirituality underscores a key point: There is a spiritual dimension to human problems and solutions" (3).

Given this reality, it makes sense that psychotherapists wish to address spirituality and religion with their clients. In an effort to treat the whole person, it is crucial that we understand the potential that spirituality and religion hold for both well-being and mental suffering.

Once again, the caution is that this approach, in isolation, does not constitute a holistic therapy. It is nonetheless a crucial aspect of holistic treatment, and traditionally categorized spiritual interventions can be very helpful in helping clients achieve mental well-being.

Mind-Body (and Spiritual-Social-Energy) Therapies

As is the case with somatic therapies, some mind-body approaches to treatment are bio-reductionist. Many such forms of therapy conceive of mind as secondary to the body. There are other holistic therapists who have created approaches based on the equal importance of mind and body, including the idea that mind can change the body. Others recognize the unity of mind, body, and spirit. Still others recognize that relationships and the social environment must be considered as part of the whole person. There is also some tentative movement toward understanding the role of energy in mental well-being.

Mind-body therapy is based on the idea that mind and body cannot be separated: altering one changes the other. According to the United States Department of Health and Human Services, mind-body therapies include tai chi, qigong, yoga, acupuncture, and meditation (National Institutes of Health National Center for Complimentary and Integrative Health n.d.). These techniques have been shown in research to help people relieve a number of physical symptoms such as pain and irritable bowel syndrome as well as some mental difficulties such as depression and anxiety. Mind-body therapies are believed to improve physical functioning through the process of altering the stress response (see, for example, Graubard, Perez-Sanchez, and Katta 2021; Jacobs 2001a; Jacobs 2001b). Likewise, a central tenet of mind-body medicine is that physical interventions (i.e., massage, the practice of yoga) can relieve mental suffering, such as the sequelae of trauma or depression or anxiety, by altering the nervous system. As you can see, they both come down to changes in the nervous system. In other words, in mind-body therapy, mind and body are one, and that one tends to end up being neurochemical. To be sure, this is not the view of every mind-body therapist, but it is the focus on most of the research and academic literature on the subject. If one is a committed materialist, then the body is real, and the mind is not. Therefore, looking primarily at the body *is* looking at the whole person. But if one holds that there is more to humanity than our bodies, then a genuinely holistic psychotherapy will certainly include focus on the body but will not be limited to it.

As we saw above, many holistic therapists emphasize the importance of the spiritual nature of the person. An example of mind-body-spirit focused therapy comes from Ben-Shahar (2012). He defined holistic psychotherapy in these terms: "The word holism (from Greek, Holos) denotes the entirety of existence. Holistic psychotherapy argues that in order to understand a system we ought to take all of its dimensions into account. Holistic approaches in therapy involve a belief that therapy should not only focus on the psychological dimensions of the person (as in talk therapy) but also consider the person's bodily and spiritual levels" (Ben-Shahar 2012, 11).

Thus, the author has identified a common theme in holistic approaches: body, mind, and spirit must all be considered in treatment. Ben-Shahar (2012) also includes the idea that the self is relational, which can be viewed on the interpersonal level and/or the transpersonal or collective level.

Mazzotta identifies as a spiritual empowerment coach, healer, and therapist. She edited a volume on holistic therapy that includes working with mind, body and spirit. Like other holistic therapists, she places emphasis on the sense of self. Like Thompson (2019, 2020, 64-71), Mazzotta has framed holistic therapy as an alternative to the medical model. This is an important aspect of holistic therapy in my view.

Mazzotta (2022) pointed out the degree to which a diagnosis of a mental illness can be iatrogenic: leaving an individual feel that they are inherently deficient. Her focus in her approach to holistic mental health treatment is to engender a sense of agency over one's life. While agency is an important aspect of well-being, we need to temper this observation with an acknowledgment that it can become a slippery slope to the degree that individualism can leave a person feeling that they should be able to fix themselves. To be clear, Mazzotta does not make that claim. Her introduction to the chapters by other holistic practitioners is rooted in the objective of helping people understand that a positive sense of self is at the heart of a good life. In chapter one, Mazzotta (2022) emphasized this point: you are worthy, and you have a purpose. The sense of self will arise repeatedly as we look at other approaches to holistic therapy.

Mazzotta's (2022) text is largely dedicated to techniques that focus on specific aspects of mental difficulties such as trauma and sense of self, which transcend diagnosis. The mix of techniques includes several somatic/body-based techniques and various forms of guided meditation/affirmation.

Another approach to psychotherapy that combines mind, body, social issues, and spirituality is Contemplative Psychotherapy (Loizzo et al. 2023). Once again, we see in this approach a heavy emphasis on neuroscience, although the authors seem to appreciate a bidirectional causation. For example, Loizzo et al. (2023) noted that mindfulness empowers the prefrontal cortex, and compassion meditations work by empowering the limbic cortex. This suggests that the author does not believe that brain *causes* mind because mind can create changes in brain physiology.

Contemplative Psychotherapy certainly includes mindfulness as well as moves beyond it to include compassion-based practices and embodied techniques such as "imagery, movement, and breath-work" (Loizzo et al. 2023, xxvi). This author noted that Contemplative Psychotherapy is more suited to address the suffering caused by harmful social forces because the treatment is not centered on a dyad (therapist and client) but is more often conducted in "groups, families, communities and institutions, and society at large" (Loizzo et al. 2023, xxvii). This theme is amplified in the chapter written by Majied (2023, 3-12). She emphasized the use of contemplative practices to combat the effects of colonialism and the value of practices created by People of the Global Majority (PGM), a less value-laden term than Black, Indigenous, People of Color (BIPOC).

Contemplative Psychotherapy draws on knowledge from a number of different disciplines. The system also embraces perspectives and practices from PGM. The Majied chapter (2023, 3-12) specifically cited nature-based and embodied practices such as drumming, chanting, and sun, earth, and water practices. We see in this system then the integration of disciplines, perspectives, and techniques as well as an emphasis on body, mind, social circumstances, and spirituality.

Edge's Eclectic Therapy

Edge's (2011) Eclectic Therapy is, in my opinion, a misnomer. She has created an approach to therapy that brings in several different techniques from several schools of therapy, but her model goes beyond technical eclecticism. Technical eclecticism is understood among therapy integrationists as a hodgepodge of techniques with no unifying or underlying logic for their combination. Theoretical integration is the creation of a new model by means of combining previously existing approaches into a cohesive unit under the aegis of a connecting logic. (Zarbo et al. 2015). Given this difference, it was surprising to me when I encountered Edge's work. Her model represents a holistic approach that brings together diverse elements based on a clear metatheoretical position.

Edge's (2011) basic premise is that clients present with a variety of needs, from pain management to anxiety reduction to finding the true self. Because clients' needs are so varied and complex, the clinician must be able to draw on elements from "philosophical, theoretical, experiential, and empirically based stances" (Edge 2011, 1). Not only do clients have a variety of needs that require disciplinary integration, the fact that people are body, mind and spirit also requires therapists to draw on diverse sources of understanding. Additionally, each client is multifaceted not only on the individual level, but they are also situated within the cosmos. Edge's (2011) approach to holistic therapy recognizes both the nature of individuals as separate entities as well as situates them in the "sea of existence that supports and sustains" (2). While symptom reduction may be the presenting problem it is typically not the final result a client desires. The goal of this treatment is wholeness. This includes the integration of the human triune nature, meeting people's multifaceted needs and awareness of their cosmic context.

Edge (2011) stressed the importance of the connection between the consciousness of the therapist and that of the client as central to the healing process. This connection shows up as "intuition, inner knowing, precognition, telepathy, and other experiences" (18). These ways of knowing are applied in the context of a humanistic and transpersonal orientation.

As a Transpersonal therapist, Edge (2011) places a good bit of emphasis on higher states of consciousness. She seeks to help clients find meaning as well as "sense something of the beyond" (3). Once again, we see that the line between spirituality and therapy is no line at all but more the center territory of a Venn diagram. She stressed her commitment to spiritual psychology. Citing the work of Robert Sardello, Edge brings the development of specific virtues into the therapy process. The virtues she advocates as appropriate objectives in treatment are devotion, balance, faithfulness, selflessness, compassion, courtesy, equanimity, patience, truth, courage, discernment, and love.

Edge (2011) included in her work an understanding of the role of energy in well-being. Energy healing has received some support in research. For example, Reiki is now considered an evidence-based adjunct treatment for both physical and emotional difficulties (Lee, Pittler and Ernst 2008). Edge (2011) referenced the Association for Comprehensive Energy Psychology (ACEP) in stating that psychological problems are "a reflection of disturbed bioenergetic patterns" (80).

As we can see, Edge's (2011) "eclectic" therapy is integrative in that several theoretical approaches are brought together with an underlying logic and worldview. It includes many of the elements of a truly holistic therapy: mind, body, spirit, relationship, and energy. The diversity of aspects of a person and issues with which they present requires not only a combination of many theoretical approaches, but also must include disciplines beyond psychology.

Thompson's HEART Model

Neil Thompson is a social worker who has critiqued the medical model as insufficient to address the mental health crisis, and has proposed a holistic approach to remedy the situation. He identified holistic as including bio-psycho-social-spiritual elements. His approach to mental well-being includes multiple disciplines, focusing specifically on symbolic interactionism in sociology and existentialism in philosophy. From existentialism, he drew out the importance of meaning as fundamental to well-being. Meaning is, in turn, related to issues of identity, roles, and power, which are social issues. These concerns can be expressed in ways that lead to alienation, which Thompson (2010, 2020, 64-71) identified as a root cause of depression, anxiety, and psychosis. Let us take a deeper look at symbolic interactionism as an element in a holistic approach to mental health.

Symbolic Interactionism

Before we look explicitly at Thompson's (2010, 2020, 64-71) use of symbolic interactionism in his holistic model, a brief look at what the term includes may be helpful. The concepts that are central to symbolic interactionism are typically credited to the philosopher G. H Meade, although the term itself was coined by Blumer in 1937, who used the term in the context of sociology. Symbolic interactionism is premised on the idea that humans are fundamentally and irreducibly social. That is, there cannot be an understanding of an individual absent an understanding of their social (and physical) environmental context (Burbank and Martins 2009).

This applies to one's sense of self or identity. A person can reflect on self-as-object as a way of formulating an understanding of themselves. But this is inextricably tied to the way that another person is interacting or has interacted with the first person.

One of the crucial contributions of Mead's theory is the insight that the emergence of the self can be understood as a result of the capacity for perspective-taking. "By looking at themselves through the eyes of others, individuals internalise [*sic*] the cultural narratives and normative standards of their groups(s), evaluate their actions accordingly, and, thereby, build up complex identities which remain dependent on their social environment and the recognition of others" (Nungesser 2021, 31).

This quote represents one moment in a reflexive arc. A person is born into a society and internalizes that society's worldview, beliefs, and norms. The narratives highly influence how the person comes to see their self. The second moment in the process is when that individual acts in the world. The action will be partially based on their identity, and it will likewise influence the cultural worldview, attitudes, and beliefs. In many cases, the individual ratifies the status quo; for example, I see myself as a woman and will act in the world in the ways women are supposed to act, thus contributing to a world in which my child is born and will likely internalize and act out a gender binary with attendant roles. Of course, this isn't always the case. We will examine that possibility later. The point here is this: according to symbolic interactionism, my identity is at least partially based on the culture that I am born into. This is partly due to the categories the culture recognizes.

As this discussion of gender may suggest, symbolic interactionists have discussed roles and the relationship between roles and status and power (Carter and Fuller 2016). Continuing with the gender example, the feminine role is granted less status and afforded less power than males are in cultures the world over. An important role in our discussion is that of physician. This role requires a reciprocal one: patient. In this binary, physicians are granted a great deal of status and power in our culture. The role of patient carries a status of dependency born out of relative ignorance. In the case of mental health, this means that psychiatric patients are seen as weak and dependent. The perspective of the psychiatrist will have more sway than alternative perspectives, and a psychiatrist's diagnosis and treatment recommendations will have more power than that of either a therapist or the patient.

As one may readily see, the concept of meaning is intimately tied to roles, power, and status. As a primary focus of symbolic interactionism, Blumer (1969) posited three basic principles regarding meaning:

1. Human beings act toward things on the basis of the meanings the things have for them.
2. The meaning of things is derived from or arises out of social interaction that one has with others.
3. These meanings are handled in and modified through an interpretative process used by the person in dealing with the things he or she encounters (Blumer 1969, 2).

Meaning is created through symbols, language being the primary symbol humans use to share meaning (Carter and Fuller 2016). Language naturalizes a great deal of meaning: by internalizing the language, one sees certain situations as natural and alternatives as unnatural and thus unacceptable or deviant. For Thompson (2019, 2020, 64-71), the understanding symbolic interactionism brings to the topic of mental health and illness is a sociological perspective that must be included in a holistic approach to address mental suffering.

Meaning

The work of the symbolic interactionists is an important element in Thompson's (2019) holistic approach to mental health. Much of the influence of culture and interpersonal interactions within the cultural context is due to the way that they influence the meaning a person holds for their experiences. Thompson stressed that we must understand how the meaning of mental illness has affected those who have been thus labeled by powerful representatives of the status quo. We must understand how it has affected their sense of self and especially how it has created a sense of alienation. In explicating this view,

Thompson (2019) has demonstrated that the dominant Western approach to mental illness has actually contributed to difficulties in living rather than clearing a way to help people move toward mental well-being.

In Thompson's (2019) explication of the role of meaning in mental illness and mental health, he augmented the work of symbolic interactionists with that of the existentialists. Existentialism posits that while life has no absolute truth that can serve as a guiding principle, we must all find meaning, value and purpose in our lives. Humans are innately meaning-making creatures. We develop meaning to make sense of our experiences. Meaning is developed in a dialectic between subject and object. That is, the individual must elaborate meaning based on their subjectivity. But as we have seen, that subjectivity is largely formed out of social interactions. This means that the sense of self is a constantly emerging property. Rather than being a fixed entity, it is a fluid process that is dependent on social interactions and context.

According to Thompson (2019), interactions are carried out by means of symbolic communication. Language is, of course, one of the central means of doing so but not the only such means. For example, one's attire or other aspects of appearance may signify a role. These symbolic markers create frames in which two people may interact. These frames, in turn, influence the meaning that one may elaborate in relation to the interaction. The frames and their attendant roles are typically associated with a power differential, such as psychiatrist and patient.

At the center of mental well-being is a sense of safety and security, which comes from being able to make sense of our experiences and have those experiences recognized as legitimate in our social context. When our experiences are contradicted or completely ignored or when meaning is imposed on one by members of more powerful groups, a sense of alienation ensues. According to Thompson (2019), alienation is at the heart of mental illness and is a result of a great deal of our current approach to mental illness.

Thompson (2019) observed that under the aegis of the medical model, mental illness is highly stigmatized. People who experience mental suffering are the victims of pejorative stereotypes and distorted perceptions. That is, they are "othered." This fuels a negative identity that leads to isolation, estrangement, a sense of inadequacy, and despair.

An important aspect of alienation is the degree to which it not only exacerbates the situation for those who suffer from a mental illness but, in fact, causes mental suffering. Anyone whose behavior or sense of self falls outside social expectations and norms is alienated. That is, the meaning one elaborates around their lives and their sense of self may fall outside the categories the language and culture has naturalized. They are seen as unnatural. This causes great psychological harm.

According to Thompson (2019), the way to help clients heal from this psychological insult is spirituality. He is clear that spirituality does not mean religious commitment. Rather, spirituality is a system of creating/assigning meaning to events and life in general. Closely associated with this meaning is direction and purpose. To achieve mental well-being, one must be able to see events and life as meaningful, and one must be able to find purpose and direction based on that meaning.

Trauma and Loss

The medical model of mental illness has focused on the individual and how mental illness is an individual phenomenon; there is some dysfunction or deficit within the person that leads to suffering. Thompson (2019) is clear that we have come a long way in realizing the degree to which interactions create mental distress. Simply put, trauma predicts mental status.

Thompson (2019) observed that, in many cases, there is a proximal trigger for an episode of mental illness. But close inspection reveals that the event was, in fact, connected to past trauma. Thus, trauma creates vulnerability to future mental difficulties, and the underlying trauma must be treated to help an individual achieve optimal functioning. This is equally true for any of the adverse childhood experiences that have been shown to contribute to future mental and physical problems. Again, it is clear in this shift from neurochemical imbalance to interpersonal interactions that the underlying cause of mental suffering is social, and the focus for treatment must include how the social context has contributed to the meaning, purpose and direction of a client's life.

Emotions

In his bio-psycho-social-spiritual approach to mental health, Thompson (2019) also stressed the role of emotions in mental suffering and well-being. He noted that under the medical model, overfocus on the brain has served to "prioritize the cognitive aspects of human psychology, while the focus on risk and public protection has tended to prioritize behavior.…The emotional dimension has therefore tended to be marginalized, pushed into a peripheral role" (Thompson 2019, xviii). He reiterated his position the following year: "'mental' health…[has] a strong focus on *cognitive* aspects (the presumed 'irrationality' of madness, for example), where what I was witnessing had much more to do with the *emotional* challenges of people's lives" (2020, 70, emphasis in original). He observed that in his work with people who were suffering from mental pain, what he experienced was that it "had more to do, figuratively speaking, with heart than with head" (70).

Conclusion: Putting it All Together: What is Holistic Therapy?

If by holistic therapy we wish to stake a territory outside the boundaries of the medical model, we must base our work on the view that a person is more than a body and their mental suffering is not a disease of the brain or reducible—let alone treatable—by simply altering the neurochemistry of the person's body. It is equally important that we see work beyond the medical model as transcending diagnostic categories and helping people resolve concerns beyond symptom reduction.

As I hope you have realized by now, the categories noted on the Verywell Mind website—somatic, spiritual, mind-body (along with spirit-social-energetic) and eclectic (integrated)—are not mutually exclusive. They overlap in many important ways and, taken together along with the HEART model create a picture of a complex approach to human suffering and healing. While some forms of therapy are labeled holistic when they are in fact bio-reductionist, this is not the general stance of holistic therapists. In some cases, when a psychotherapist offers an adjunct to talk therapy that is somatically focused—like trauma-aware yoga, or if they offer a technique that is associated with a form of spirituality or religion, like meditation, or practices a form of therapy that integrates several different schools—they may brand themselves as holistic. I am suggesting that the use of techniques that fall outside the aegis of standard talk therapy is not enough to qualify a practitioner as holistic. Thompson's work (2019, 2020, 64-71) reminds us that while biological, psychological, and spiritual issues are very important, we must remain aware of the social aspects of mental suffering. As Edge (2011) and Majied (2023, 3-12) have suggested, holistic psychotherapy is the understanding of multiple disciplines and cultural perspectives, along with the integration of several schools of therapy, all unified by means of an overarching theory and metatheory that holds the multiple pieces together to form an approach. While I am not advocating that there is a singular overarching metatheory or theory that qualifies one as holistic, a holistic practitioner must have a unifying metatheory.

This is part of the greatness of holistic therapy: it transcends the schoolism that Duval et al. (1999) have recognized as parochial and unhelpful. I am, however, an advocate of having a metatheory and theory that creates an environment in which a therapist can improvise. For this reason, I prefer to work with a basic understanding of questions like "what is mind?" and "what is the relationship between mind and body?" How does mental suffering come about? What helps move a person from mental suffering to well-being? It is with a desire to work with a clear view of these issues that I developed the mind-centered approach to therapy, which is also a holistic approach. Before we delve into this way of doing therapy, let's look at two very clearly developed forms of holistic psychology: Psychosynthesis and integral psychology. We will see that the mind-centered approach has a great deal in common with both of these orientations to therapy as well as some important differences.

Holistic Practice Points

- Holistic therapy understands a person to be a whole composed of many parts. Among these parts are their mind, their body, their spirit, their social environment, and their energy or energetic field. Assess, explore, and process with your client all these aspects of their functioning.
- In order to address the whole person, several different disciplines, theories, and techniques can be utilized in therapy. Some of the techniques are not traditionally viewed as psychological interventions. Some techniques are taken from Eastern and Indigenous healing practices. Techniques are used based on the needs of the individual client. Use your continuing education to learn different theoretical orientations. There are hundreds of forms of therapy today. Consider how different approaches fit within your metatheory of help/healing.
- Avail yourself of continuing education that introduces alternative healing techniques, such as the use of tarot in psychotherapy, trauma-informed yoga, Reiki or other energy healing systems, shamanic journeying, and others. The list is nearly infinite. Find what resonates with your individual client.
- Sociology must be included in the list of disciplines that inform our work.

- Explore with clients the ways that social structures and interactions contribute to their identity and how this affects their mental health.

- One of the more profound negative impacts of the social structure is the effects of power differentials in society and the ways that these lead to alienation. Help your client identify how or if they have been situated in social categories and the roles they have been assigned. Explore how this affects their sense of self and their quality of life.

- Helping clients develop meaning is key to their well-being. This includes the need to help them find direction and purpose in their lives. This is the spiritual aspect of psychotherapy.

- Trauma and loss often play an originating role in suffering (that is, external forces rather than purely intrapsychic functioning are at the heart of much mental illness). Explore any sources of trauma and adverse childhood experiences as well as how current relationships may have adverse effects on your clients' well-being.

- Holistic psychotherapy must have an underlying logic by means of which multiple perspectives can be combined. I am not advocating that all holistic therapists hold the same underlying logic but simply that they all have an underlying logic. Spend time contemplating what you believe the nature of reality is, what it means to be human, and what healing is. Again, avail yourself of alternative perspectives. A good place to start may be to read about materialism and post-materialist worldviews.

Chapter Four

Psychosynthesis

One of the points made in the last chapter was that holistic therapy is more than a grab bag of techniques or theories. Instead, to be truly holistic, a therapeutic approach should form a cohesive whole based on a unifying theory or metatheory. In this chapter and the next, we will look at two holistic psychotherapies that have particularly well-developed metatheoretical and theoretical foundations. We will see that the two different theoretical formulations are both supported by a well-articulated metatheory that is post-materialist. Holistic therapy aims beyond symptom reduction or the treatment of mental illnesses. Psychosynthesis holds that human well-being reaches a peak upon self-realization or apprehending the transcendent nature of the Self.

Roberto Assagioli began to develop Psychosynthesis in 1911. He also used the term bio-psychosynthesis for his holistic approach to achieve self-realization. Assagioli himself was a person of wide-ranging interests. As a psychiatrist and trained psychoanalyst, he was very interested in helping people overcome mental suffering (Nocelli 2021). And as will become clear through this discussion, Psychosynthesis places a high premium on spiritual concerns in helping clients achieve this end. As Assagioli held a primary interest in somatic disorders, he was acutely aware of the relationship between the mind and the body.

He—and particularly later disciples—also recognized the social applications of Psychosynthesis.

As a spiritual approach, we will see that the goal of Psychosynthesis is self-realization that far transcends the amelioration of psychiatric symptoms. Likewise, Psychosynthesis integrates or unifies several forms of therapy but also, and more importantly, several disciplines. There is a focus on the self in Psychosynthesis as well as on various levels of consciousness. We will also see that Psychosynthesis uses the concept of energy to a highly developed degree. These are themes that we have noted in the previous chapter, which are brought together by a post-materialist metatheory. Thus, we will learn that Psychosynthesis is a bio-psycho-social-spiritual-energetic approach to mental well-being.

Integration of Disciplines and Therapeutic Models

Holistic approaches to psychotherapy share the characteristic of being integrated approaches. And indeed, the synthesis in Psychosynthesis means both the synthesis of different ways of understanding humanity as well as a synthesis of diverse aspects of processes within the individual. Assagioli ([1965] 2012) was clear that his integrated approach was "systematic," as opposed to being "mere eclecticism." In insisting on systematic integration, he was clear that there must be a "specific plan of the treatment…directed towards [*sic.*] clearly envisioned aims" (6). In other words, there must be an underlying logic or theoretical foundation to give the model coherence.

Today, the breadth of learning of Roberto Assagioli would be considered unusual as he pursued a degree in medicine as well as held interests in literature and spirituality. He was a psychiatrist who was involved in an avant-garde literary group that disparaged the positivism and materialism of the natural sciences. He studied with Jung and later with Freud. He also studied Sanskrit and Eastern mysticism and was involved with the Theosophical Society. Later in his life, he studied progressive Judaism (Nocelli 2021). Given these activities, one should not be surprised that he began to look at a system that was both psychologically and spiritually focused, and he integrated knowledge from the sciences and the humanities from Western and Eastern perspectives. As noted above, his integration was at the level of both forms of therapy as well as different "contributions to the knowledge of human nature and betterment" (Assagioli [1965] 2012, 12). He identified psychosomatic medicine; the psychology of religion; investigations of superconscious or cosmic consciousness; psychical research and parapsychology; Eastern psychology; Smuts's holistic approach (more biological than psychological but gave a prominent place to energy); the psychology of the personality; interindividual and social psychology; and various active techniques as areas of knowledge incorporated into Psychosynthesis (Assagioli [1965] 2012).

In Psychosynthesis, the metatheory is more implied than overt. Hopefully, it will be clear as we work through the theory that psychosynthesists hold that consciousness (or mind) is real and fundamental. We will see that while body is important in this approach, consciousness, spirit, and energy are the loci of attention. We will also see that the relationship between the practitioner and client is an important aspect of treatment.

The Self and the Unconscious

Bringing these diverse areas of study together is aimed at a singular goal in Psychosynthesis: to build a new unifying center around which we create a coherent, organized, and unified personality (Assagioli [1965] 2012; Nocelli 2022). Assagioli referred to this end-state as Self-Realization. Human psychological suffering is viewed in this system as a result of lost unity. Unity, or self-realization, is achieved by confronting the unknown within the self. The unknown is the unconscious. Psychosynthesis understands there to be various levels of the unconscious, all of which must be confronted to achieve integration, which brings psychological well-being and transcendence.

More in keeping with Jung than Freud, Assagioli understood consciousness to be comprised of a lower unconscious, a middle unconscious, wherein awareness/consciousness resides, and a higher unconscious. All of these are nested within the collective unconscious.

The personality in Psychosynthesis is symbolized as an egg that is divided into three equal parts. The field of consciousness with the "I" is in the center third of the egg. The "I" is the lowercase s self, not unlike the Jungian notion of the ego. The bottom third of the egg is the lower unconscious. The upper third is the higher unconscious. This is the transpersonal, spiritual dimension. At the apex of the egg is the Higher Self. The egg rests within the Collective Unconscious.

The "I," or self, is the sense of personal identity (Nocelli 2021). Assagioli ([1965] 2012) is clear that the "I" is not comprised of the *contents* of identity, but it is the *awareness* of identity. As the self and the Self are closely related, we will look at this construct in more detail below. The ego-self is located in the center of the field of consciousness. This is all that most people are aware of at any given moment.

The various levels of the unconscious are seen in Psychosynthesis as being imbued with energy. When an unconscious complex is analyzed and disintegrates, there is a release of energy from that level of the unconscious. There are also latent tendencies within the self that represent a dynamic shifting of energy. These tendencies are dynamic in that they are continually changing form from emotions and impulses to become actions, imagination, or intellectual activity. In the same way, imagination can become action. Assagioli ([1965] 2012) likened the process of this shifting of energy to the alchemical process. In so doing, he called for a science of psychological energies. Many of the psychosynthetic techniques are aimed at shifting this energy within the self. The end of Psychosynthesis is marked by the coordination and subordination of the energy of the self. Given the role of will in Psychosynthesis, we may hypothesize that this latter state is due to a large degree by the power of the will.

The specific level of unconscious that dominates within an individual will determine what kinds of experiences and difficulties in living they will face. The lower unconscious is identified with the Freudian unconscious. This is where drives, urges, and instincts reside. This is also the domain of repressed experiences. Energy from the lower unconscious can give rise to uncontrolled parapsychological experiences and pathological symptoms such as anxiety and paranoia (Assagioli [1965] 2012). When the lower unconscious energies flow up to affect the field of consciousness, the "I" becomes overfocused on issues of security and safety. Yet it is important to note that the energy from the lower unconscious is not entirely negatively valanced. The energy of the lower unconscious provides the individual with playfulness and spontaneity, and these features must be developed and integrated.

The middle unconscious is comprised of all the things an individual does not need to be aware of in the current moment. These are things like self-esteem, self-image, higher emotions, rational beliefs, and values (Sorensen 2016). When the "I" is overidentified with the middle nonconscious, the individual experiences difficulties around the issue of identity.

The higher unconscious is the source of intuition and inspiration, love, and ecstasy (Assagioli [1965] 2012). When one is energized by the higher unconscious, there is an expanded identity. This leads to a movement toward deeper meaning and purpose and life (Sorensen 2016).

Above the higher unconscious is the Higher Self. Sorensen (2016) used the term "soul" for this aspect of the personality. It is also referred to as the Transpersonal Self. This features the ability to recognize oneself as part of a unified singularity without losing individual uniqueness.

The Higher Self is connected to the ego "I"/self. The ego-self is at the center of the field of awareness (in the middle unconscious) and is a projection of the Higher Self. Sorensen (2016) referred to it as a "contraction" of the Self. It is the "mind's need to limit and isolate itself…to separate itself from its surroundings" (34). This "I" can be fed by the energies of the three different levels of unconscious. But when it becomes connected to the Higher Self, the duality between the two dissolves. One realizes one's true nature as a participatory element in the divine.

The entire egg is surrounded by the collective unconscious. There is no strict division between the Collective Unconscious and the personality. In fact, all levels or areas of the egg are permeable. Nocelli (2021) divided the collective unconscious into three areas as well. The lower collective unconscious is the seat of the primitive, archaic collective unconscious. Much of this is included in the archetypes from humanity's past. The middle collective unconscious contains contents from the present sociocultural situation. The higher collective unconscious contains the future potential of humanity and is integrative, evolutionary, and synthetic (Nocelli 2021).

The Will and Other Psychic Functions

The way we become aware of and utilize the unconscious energies of the personality is through an act of will. The will is of central importance to Psychosynthesis. The will is the central psychic function. Assagioli ([1965] 2012) gave credit to Jung for identifying four functions within the personality. For Jung, the personality was one's way of making sense of the world. The way that one typically experiences is based on four functions that are two sets of binaries. One tends to depend more on thinking or feeling to make sense of life; likewise, one has a tendency to use sensations or intuition. In Psychosynthesis, the psychological functions are understood to be abilities with which we act on the world. To function optimally, one ultimately should be able to use all of the abilities.

Assagioli saw Jung's list of psychological functions as partial. He offered a six-pointed star symbol. The star symbol captures the sense of radiating energy. The center of the star is the will, which is a regulating function (Nocelli 2021). It directs energy through intention

(Sorensen 2016) and helps one formulate goals, deliberate on options, make decisions, and make and execute plans. While we may tend to think of the will as imposing or coercive, authentic will brings a sense of liberation and freedom. It is the ability to choose, including "what meaning we give to our existence and what attitude we chose to cultivate towards (*sic)* events in our lives" (Nocelli, 70). The will is the center of one's power; with power comes responsibility.

Radiating out from the will are six abilities. The bottom ray represents sensation. This is associated with embodiment. The bottom ray energizes the body with the life force that is necessary for health. The ray to the left of sensation is feeling. Feeling brings the ability to give valence to experience: we can discern if something is comfortable or uncomfortable, desirable or undesirable. It is the basic approach-avoidance reaction necessary for survival. It is the seat of information from within our bodies and from the external world. To the right of the bottom ray is desire. Desire includes the ability to discern and use "instincts, drives, wishes, needs, attractions and repulsions" (Sorensen 2016, 50). The ray that points upward is intuition. Remember that intuition is an energy that emanates from the higher unconscious. Although it is essentially transpersonal, Assagioli placed it in the group of functions because it is available even to those who are not identified with the higher unconscious energies (Sorensen 2016). It helps us realize our interconnectedness, and this interconnectedness provides access to information from beyond us. To the left of intuition is imagination. Our imaginative ability is our ability to create. Sorensen (2016) associated imagination with our ability to visualize, although we are capable of imagining in a multitude of ways. Sorensen made the point that imagination is "real" and has the ability to influence our lives to a high degree. Finally, to the right of intuition is thought. Thought is the interpretive function. In thinking, we can collect, organize, label and categorize information (Sorensen 2016). It is the linear, discursive, problem-solving capacity.

Development

For Assagioli ([1965] 2012), human suffering is the result of feeling divided. There is an unarticulated yearning for our original unity but a pervasive feeling of separation. As a result, people neither know nor understand themselves and therefore lack self-control. This brings about mental suffering: despair, discouragement, and doubt. This, in turn, propels us into frenetic activity (which includes emotional instabilities) as a form of escape.

The way out of this mire is to achieve "harmonious integration" (Assagioli [1965] 2012, 18). It is true self-realization that necessarily includes harmony with others. This process unfolds in nonlinear stages. The first stage is to achieve awareness of one's personality. This means bringing material from the lower level of the unconscious into awareness. We must discover the "dark forces" and conflicts that dominate us. For Assagioli, the method to uncover this material is psychoanalysis. Assagioli ([1965] 2012) stressed that the analyst must be objective and impartial in the process, meaning that they should refrain from imposing their theoretical bias—in other words, to engage in analysis with evenly hovering attention (in the words of Freud) or without memory or desire (in the words of Bion).

The second stage toward psychic freedom is to learn to control the elements of the personality. Assagioli ([1965] 2012) noted that "We are dominated by everything with which our self becomes identified. We can dominate and control everything from which we disidentify ourselves" (19). We identify with our weaknesses, our faults, and our fears. We define and limit ourselves by our undesirable aspects. The antidote is to look for the origins of these negative self-definitions, predict their negative effects on our lives, and come to see that these self-assessments are not true. He calls this process "disidentification." Again, Assagioli stressed the debt to psychoanalysis. He noted that through psychoanalysis, we have learned that unconscious conflicts and dynamics exert a great deal of power over one's life as long as they remain unconscious. But when they are brought to the light of awareness, they can be understood and lose their grip on a person. The degree to which one is able to observe with some distance these unconscious contents, the more one is able to realize the fundamental untruth of them. The energy that has been locked in these unconscious dynamics is released and can be controlled and directed into pursuits of one's choosing. In Psychosynthesis, the point of bringing material from the lower unconscious into the field of consciousness is to use the energy thus released for constructive purposes.

The third step in the process of self-realization is to discover the unifying center of the self or realize the True Self. An intermediate step in this process is to create new identifications. This can mean the creation of an ideal model. This begins by examining our various self-images (Nocelli 2021). Put differently, we identify our different subpersonalities or parts. After disidentifying with those that do not serve us, we experience the "I"—the observer. Then we create a model that will serve as an inspiration. By applying will, this aspirational image becomes manifest and embodied, to be lived out and thus transform our daily life. In other words, based on the directed use of imagination, we cultivate an attitude based on self-knowledge and clarity of purpose (Nocelli 2021). This attitude is not yet another false self, based on role expectations or the needs of others. It is a projection of one's center into the world. This new way of being in the world is a connection between the "I" and the higher Self. One's higher Self is projected into and symbolized by the new lived experience of the "I."

The last stage of the developmental process outlined by Psychosynthesis is true Psychosynthesis: the personality coalesces around a new center, one that is coherent, organized, and unified. It is, again, not an idealized image that is not authentic but a dynamic, creative concentration of energy. This widens the channel of communication with the higher Self. The construction of the new personality moves in three parts. First, one learns how to use available energies. Energies become available when unconscious complexes are disintegrated, much like how the dismantling of an atom releases energy. One can also tap into latent tendencies that have hitherto been neglected. This is a process of transmutation from thought to feeling or feeling to imagination, etc. The second phase is the development of the underdeveloped aspects of the personality. Just as calisthenics can build muscle, exercises can build mental capacities for memory, imagination, and will. Finally, mental energies and functions are coordinated and subordinated to the will so that the personality is organized.

Mutative Functions in Psychosynthesis

There are three main healing techniques in Psychosynthesis. As has already been noted, Assagioli was trained as an analyst and utilized analytic techniques to discover and dissolve unconscious conflicts and dynamisms that contribute to mental suffering. The role of the relationship between the psychosynthesizer and client is also important and mutative in and of itself. But Psychosynthesis is primarily an experiential process, and so the bulk of the interventions in Psychosynthesis is the use of various techniques aimed at helping clients have certain experiences.

In Psychosynthesis, there is a large value placed on the psychosynthesist having achieved their own self-realization before they attempt to lead others through the process. Techniques can only be appropriately applied by one who has found their true center. This is partly due to the action of "spontaneous irradiation" (Nocelli 2021, 92). This is the "inevitable influence of the therapist" (204). This influence is always present. It is always occurring as a flow of energy but can be consciously directed by the therapist through intention: the "will-to-good, the act of blessing" (205). This intention occurs in the context of the Rogerian core conditions and a guiding relationship that is centered on human respect and free of directive or prescriptive features.

The stress on the therapist remaining nondirective and nonprescriptive is particularly important in relation to the many techniques that Psychosynthesis utilizes. Assagioli ([1965] 2012) noted, "In Psychosynthesis the emphasis is put on a holistic or integral conception of the treatment… to which every method, exercise and technique should be subordinated. The needs not only of each patient but also of the different phases of the treatment in each case are very different and sometimes opposite. Therefore, the use of a specific technique or exercise which may prove useful in one case or in one phase may be unsuitable or even harmful for other individuals or in different conditions" (59).

Having stated that, the majority of the literature produced by psychosynthesists is focused on various exercises to help clients directly experience disidentification and synthesis. Clients are asked to write, including journaling, and to engage in a host of guided meditations or active imagination exercises. The therapist can suggest exercises in drawing, clay modeling, and listening to and/or performing music. Hypnosis (in terms of direct suggestion in a light trance) can be used in Psychosynthesis. Various body techniques are also used (Nocelli 2021).

The Role of Spirituality

Psychosynthesis unfolds in two phases or on two levels: personal Bio-psychosynthesis and transpersonal Psychosynthesis (Nocelli 2022). The personal level of Psychosynthesis is not as overtly spiritual as the transpersonal level. Indeed, on the more personal level of Psychosynthesis, more psychoanalytic techniques are used to pursue the very psychoanalytic goal of making unconscious conflicts and dynamics conscious. Personal Psychosynthesis moves beyond this, however, in that once the unconscious material is exhumed, the focus shifts to organizing the biological and psychological elements around the personal self. Once the personal self has a new center, when we are able to make choices and live our ideal (to be explored below), one may choose to move toward transpersonal Psychosynthesis.

Transpersonal Psychosynthesis is concerned with more spiritual pursuits. The process culminates with the manifestation of superconscious forces (Nocelli 2022). This can be achieved in one of two ways. Either the personal self, or "I," ascends toward the higher Self, or one opens oneself to the energies of the higher unconscious and the higher Self (Nocelli 2022). That is, these energies descend to the "I," altering it. Either process (ascension or descension toward union of the "I" and the Higher Self) may culminate in a form of awakening or illumination or realization of the transpersonal Self.

Assagioli was insistent that Psychosynthesis was not aligned with any particular religion. He was likewise clear that his system is based on the assumption of the existence of a divine intelligence that expresses itself in humans as the drive to love (Sorensen 2016). Assagioli had a good bit of experience with Buddhist philosophy and practice as well associations with the Theosophical Society and with Judaism (Nocelli 2021). Yet he eschewed the word "spiritual" in relation to Psychosynthesis, preferring the term "transpersonal" as more neutral and scientific (Nocelli 2022). While Psychosynthesis is not about pursuing mystical experiences or pursuing any specific metaphysical commitment, it is centered on the notion that the body is the channel through which spiritual energies manifest on earth (Sorensen 2016).

Biological Considerations

It may be clear that Assagioli was focused on the psyche: the mind and the spirit. But for Assagioli, harmonization of the personality included awareness of the relationship between our bodies and our inner life (Salvini 2022, 321-339). According to Salvini, because our bodies are concrete while our Higher Selves are more abstract, the perception of the body may be easier to accomplish than that of the Self. The tangible nature of the body allows us to begin to see the connections between parts, to see a whole made up of different pieces. This begins the process of understanding the way that multiple other parts of our selves fit together as a singularity. Our perceptions of our bodies have a powerful impact on our emotions, thoughts, behaviors, and personality. Not only does our body shape our experiences, but we must use our bodies to set the conditions for our spiritual quest. As the Higher

Self cannot be reached in a state of chaos, confusion, or clamor, we can still our bodies to quiet the mind, thus opening the channel to the Higher Self.

Social Considerations

The social aspects of Psychosynthesis are less well developed than the psychological, spiritual, energetic, or biological. One can argue that the basic belief of interconnectedness within a unified singularity has important social implications: if we are all connected, what happens to the individual affects everyone and everything. Beyond this most basic connection, Assagioli ([1965] 2012) has argued that Psychosynthesis is fruitfully used in education and interpersonal and group relationships "which sorely need to be adjusted and harmonized" (7).

Brown (2022, 421-432) has identified the use of Psychosynthesis to help communities, governments, and socioeconomic systems and climate change. She identified four ways that Psychosynthesis can help heal the current social and ecological turmoil. First, as individuals heal through Psychosynthesis, they will more readily engage in social-ecological causes. Second, Psychosynthesis may address the trauma that has already occurred and will continue to occur as a result of climate change. Third, psychosynthesists can support activists by strengthening their courage, compassion, and connection. Finally, Psychosynthesis will aid in a shift in consciousness that must occur if humanity is to survive.

An Energy Psychology

Sorensen (2016) has specifically identified Psychosynthesis as an energy healing method. References to energy and the movement and release of energy have appeared repeatedly in this chapter. We have seen that the release and movement of energies—from unconscious conflicts and dynamics, between levels of unconscious, from the will to the other abilities, and in terms of transmutation of psychological functions (like from imagination to thought, etc.)—are important in Psychosynthesis.

There are a number of forms of energy healing today. One repeated aspect that is common to various energy healing systems is the notion of the power of intention (Zahourak 2020). Intention may play a role in Psychosynthesis in the form of will. We have seen the central role of will in Psychosynthesis. Will may be another way of discussing intention. We have seen the role of intentions in the process of spontaneous irradiation in terms of the will-to-good. This poses an interesting area for further thought and study. I leave it as food for thought. I have indicated repeatedly that holistic therapy works from a bio-psycho-social-spiritual-energetic perspective.

Conclusion

Psychosynthesis is a bio-psycho-social-spiritual-energetic approach to the treatment of human suffering. The goal of Psychosynthesis is to integrate the self as well as integrate the self with the Self. The theme of integration is consistent between the goals of treatment as well as the methods and theories that can be used to achieve the goals. We see, therefore, a clear, consistent, overarching theoretical perspective that links different approaches into a unified whole. Assagioli and his followers have created a holistic approach to mental well-being that is very different from the medical model. Difficulties in living are not seen as easily divided into diagnostic categories, nor are symptoms the focus of treatment. In this system, consciousness is understood to be a key aspect of the world and of the human being. Consciousness exists both within and beyond the person and therefore beyond the brain. This post-materialist metatheory forms the foundation of a view of a multifaceted yet unified universe and a multifaceted yet unified individual. The principle of unity in multiplicity on every level allows one to see—and use—the unity in the multiplicity of disciplines relevant to human functioning and theories of psychotherapy.

Psychosynthesis has many of the elements that we saw in the last chapter on holistic therapies. One of the primary reasons this holistic approach to therapy has warranted a chapter of its own is because of the degree of theoretical elaboration that holds together the various aspects of the approach. One of the important elements is the fact that it is an integrated approach to mental well-being. While the first phase of Psychosynthesis, or personal synthesis, is primarily psychoanalytic, the second stage transcends any one therapeutic approach. The integration in Psychosynthesis is primarily comprised of a number of different disciplines that approach the human condition from different perspectives.

Psychosynthetic work occurs on the levels of the conscious and the unconscious. One of the features of Psychosynthesis is the degree to which the nature or geography of the unconscious is mapped out, with different realms of the unconscious being associated with different aspects of mental health and mental suffering.

Assagioli and his followers have placed the human will at the center of psychological functions. As an elaboration of Jung's work, the pyschosynthesists understand the will as the energetic center of the psychological functions. These include sensation, feeling, desire, intuition, imagination, and thought. Each of these functions must function optimally for mental well-being.

Assagioli understood development to be movement toward psychological unity. Unity brings self-control, which is the antidote for emotional instability. Development, from this perspective, is toward integration. This includes integration of the contents of the lower unconscious into awareness. It also means bringing under control the forces with which we have disidentified and our negative self-definitions. The third stage of development is the achievement of self-realization through identifying those parts that serve us and disidentifying with those that do not. Finally, one may achieve true synthesis to achieve a dynamic, organized, unified center.

In Psychosynthesis, there are three key mutative activities. On the most basic level, psychoanalytic techniques are employed to resolve unconscious conflicts. In addition, the therapist's mind exerts an effect on the client's mind. The therapist's energy, carried by intention, affects the client. Finally, Psychosynthesis has developed a number of techniques that are applied differentially to the client's unique needs. These cover the gamut from work in a light trance state to forms of expressive therapy to body techniques.

One may understand Psychosynthesis to be highly spiritual in orientation, but this is not Assagioli's understanding of his work. Psychosynthesis is ultimately aimed at a form of realization of the transpersonal Self. Having stated this apparently spiritual pursuit, the system is not aligned with any particular religion or spiritual system.

While the biological aspects of being human are not denied, they are not the main consideration in this holistic approach to well-being. The body must be attended to for the purpose of clearing the path toward reaching the transpersonal Self.

Finally, Psychosynthesis is an energy psychology. There is a great deal of emphasis on what and how energy is stored and released. I would like to gently suggest that this is an aspect of holistic therapies in general that is often alluded to but has not been developed to as high a degree as other aspects of human functioning.

As this overview suggests, Psychosynthesis is a well-formed theoretical perspective that brings together the psychological and spiritual aspects of human functioning. There is less emphasis on the social aspects of well-being and a step toward an understanding of energetic aspects of being human. We are beginning to see that holistic treatments combine different amounts of five ingredients: the psychological, the spiritual, the social, the biological, and the energetic. Let's hold these factors in mind as we look at another well-developed theory of holistic therapy: integral theory.

Holistic Practice Points

- While biology and psychology are important, other disciplines are needed to help people achieve well-being. As stated in the last chapter, avail yourself to learning from the humanities and social sciences.

- Psychology and spirituality are not separate. Introspect on your feelings about the relationship between psychology and spirituality, and confront any reasons you may hold for avoiding talking about spirituality in therapy.

- The sense of self is a central concern for well-being. Explore clients' sense of self, including all of the words that are hyphenated with self, like self-esteem, self-concept, self-agency, self-awareness, etc. Much of this is unconscious, so utilizing techniques that help clients access aspects of their sense of self in a relaxed, slightly altered state of consciousness is very helpful.

- There are multiple aspects or parts of self that must be integrated to achieve well-being. Unification and integration of the split self is key. Explore self states, archetypes, parts, etc. with clients. This means reading about Psychoanalytic, Jungian, and Internal Family Systems forms of therapy.

- The developmental process is a nonlinear progression toward more inclusive awareness. The pinnacle of the process is realization of the true Self. Learn developmental theories. Help clients access true Self by using various states of consciousness.

- There are multiple levels of consciousness, all of which are important to well-being. We explore unconscious material that has been rejected and repressed as well as superconscious awareness through meditation, self-hypnosis, and other methods to access altered states of consciousness.

- The will (or intentionality) is important in achieving well-being. Helping clients accept and access their will is important, particularly for those who have been taught that their will should be subverted.

- Disidentification, or moving away from defining oneself in limited ways, is equally important. Helping your clients access Self beyond ego is an important element in holistic therapy.
- The techniques are nondirective and nonprescriptive and oriented toward the experiential. Help your clients have experiences from which they learn about themselves and their Self rather than trying to convince them with logic.
- Energy is important to well-being. For clients who are comfortable doing so, you can help them become aware of and direct their energy.
- The psychosynthesist must be highly integrated to do this work. You must do your work. Holistic therapy is not for everyone. It takes a great deal of extra knowledge and experience to be adept at working in this manner.

Chapter Five

Integral Yoga, Philosophy, Psychology, and Psychotherapy

Both Edge (2011) and Assagioli ([1965] 2012) were clear that simply utilizing multiple schools of therapy or multiplying techniques aimed at psychological, somatic, spiritual, social, or energetic change is not sufficient to make treatment holistic. To be truly holistic, one needs, in Assagioli's terms, systematic integration. This is not far from the definition of what constitutes a bona fide therapy in the common factors research. There must be a well-articulated, coherent, cohesive theoretical foundation that serves to unify diverse elements. I am not suggesting here that there must be a single agreed-upon theory or metatheory held in common by all holistic therapists. I am suggesting that holistic therapists must have a coherent, cohesive theoretical/metatheoretical perspective. We see in integral theory perhaps the most well-developed and explicit metatheory among holistic therapists.

Before integral theory was a psychotherapeutic approach, it was a philosophy/yoga developed by Sri Aurobindo. Drawing on his Western education and Eastern heritage, he posited nothing less than the nature of the universe and the relationship between the human mind and the universe. Aurobindo's philosophy was taken up by a psychologist Haridas Chaudhuri, who posited a theory on the origins of mental suffering, the way to overcome suffering, and the nature of the self.

This work was, in turn, taken up by Brant Cortright, who articulated a metatheory for integrating various schools of therapy to achieve a coherent holistic approach to psychotherapy.

Ken Wilber also used Aurobindo's integral philosophy as a basis for his psychological theories. In his view, the development of the mind is key to overcoming individual and social suffering. Mark Forman, like Cortright, elaborated this psychology as a form of psychotherapy with a clear understanding of how and why various therapeutic modalities can target needs at different stages of development.

Integral refers to elements that are necessary parts of a whole. Integral philosophy, psychology, and psychotherapy thus blend various seemingly diverse elements as parts of a singular whole. Integral thinkers see the necessity to embrace Eastern and Western philosophies and psychologies, mind and matter, objectivity and subjectivity, the spiritual and the mundane, and individuality and universality. All of these aspects of the human condition must be balanced in order to live a life with depth and meaning.

Sir Aurobindo: Integral Philosophy/Yoga

Sri Aurobindo Ghose (1872–1950) was of Indian descent and raised principally in England. He studied philosophy at Cambridge University. After his time at Cambridge, he returned to India where he studied yoga and become involved in the Indian independence movement (McDermott 2001). He ultimately synthesized these apparently different interests—philosophy and politics, Western philosophy and Eastern philosophy/spirituality—into a system he interchangeably called integral philosophy and integral yoga. Philosophy—the precursor of Western psychology—and yoga both deal intimately with the nature and development of the mind. So while Aurobindo did not directly address psychology in his public writings (Cornelissen 2018) his integral thought was the basis for an integral psychology and later different forms of Integral Psychotherapy. These different aspects of Aurobindo's thought are the focus of this chapter.

Aurobindo had two major meditative experiences. In the first, he touched the impersonal non-dual Brahman, or non-Being. This is a well-documented experience among Eastern mystics. As he continued his practice, he arrived at the realization that non-Being gives rise to the universe. The material world is nothing other than the force of non-Being. Aurobindo coined the term "integral" to point to this truth and used it in two contexts: integral yoga and integral consciousness (Banerji 2012). Integral consciousness refers to his insights concerning the integrated nature of the impersonal non-dual Brahman as well as the personal, dynamic manifestation of the divine as the universe. Integral yoga is the process of psychological integration.

The singular universe exists in two moments: involution and evolution. The non-dual aspect of Consciousness manifests itself in the process of involution. "Involved" here means that it is a necessary inherent part of all that exists. Thus, non-Being is involved in the world; it is within all. Because all that exists is the Ultimate or Divine in nature, it naturally evolves or continually moves toward awareness of/ expression of the Ultimate. Aurobindo taught that humans were the highest form of consciousness on earth and that they would continue to evolve toward even higher levels of consciousness until they achieved Superconsciousness. Part of this process includes appreciation of both our necessary and precious separateness, uniqueness, and individuality as well as our oneness and inherent connectedness. It includes both the disciplines aimed at communion with the divine and work in this world aimed at uplifting humanity.

This is the foundation of Aurobindo's view of mind. He predicted David Chalmer's (1995) "hard question" of consciousness in observing that from the Western materialistic perspective, there is no satisfactory answer to the question of how mind and soul arise from inconscient matter. As we see in his theory of involution/evolution, his solution is that consciousness/mind/soul has been conjoined with matter from the beginning. From this, he arrived at the conclusion that Western objective methods of study are important. But they cannot be comprehensive as they are materialistic and blinker half of the nature of reality. Mind and matter are equally fundamental: mind is not an epiphenomenon of neural activity or the brain. To understand the nonmaterial, we must use the subjective methods of introspection and contemplation (Medhananda, 2021)

According to Aurobindo, it is the simultaneous materiality and nonmateriality of the human that causes what we recognize in the West as psychological suffering. In fact, the nonmaterial aspect of the human is both mind and spirit. Thus, the human is a tripartite creature: they are simultaneously material, mental, and spiritual. He observed, "If our existence were of one piece…there would be nothing to perplex us.…But the existence of man is a triple we, a thing mysteriously physical, mental and spiritual at once, and he knows not what are the true relations of these things" (Ghose 2001, 133).

Aurobindo's integral yoga is a process of integrating these seemingly disparate parts. In doing so, he draws upon a number of different Indian spiritual traditions. The process culminates in the "supermind." The supermind is characterized by "integral consciousness" (Banerji 2012). That is, integral yoga is the "process of integration which completes itself…in the structure of an 'integral consciousness'" (Banerji 2012, 89). And here we arrive at one of the contributions Sri Aurobindo has made to psychology. Freud and Jung concerned themselves with the difference between what we are aware of and able to reflect on—the conscious—from that which we are unaware of but nonetheless affects our mental life and personality to a high degree—the unconscious. Likewise, Aurobindo explicated the nature of consciousness and the unconscious (Sen 2018).

Thus, like Freud and Jung, the psychological process that Aurobindo was describing was the process of making the unconscious conscious in order to be integrated and thus harmonize the personality (Sen 2018). In Aurobindo's psychology, there are three concentric systems of the human personality: the outer, the inner, and the inmost or true nature (Cornelissen 2020). The outer system is the normal waking state, equivalent to the Freudian notion of the conscious. The inner system includes ranges both below (roughly equivalent to the Freudian unconscious) and above normal waking consciousness. In going above normal waking consciousness, the inner system goes well beyond the Freudian concept. It is more, not less connected to others and the world and has broader and higher ranges of experience. The inmost or true nature is Self: "transcendent, immutable, and eternal" (Cornelissen 2020, 89).

The point of practice in this system is to bring order to chaos. In our ordinary waking consciousness, we are unaware of how the cacophony of needs, desires, tastes, and so forth pull us in conflicting directions and give rise to suffering. In bringing awareness to unconscious material, we are able to bring order to these diverse impulses. We can reach beyond the ego and achieve harmony within and between ourselves and the universe.

To accomplish this, one allows the contents of the unconscious to break into consciousness along with the further intention of giving the unconscious material coherence. Put differently, one must engage in the process with a strong will for becoming integrated (Sen 2018). Along with the intention, one adopts a dispassionate attitude toward the unconscious contents, for to approach them without some distance would bolster the process of repression or suppression. From this superconscious perch, one is able to view the unconscious and bring it into harmony with the personality.

Haridas Chaudhuri: Integral Yoga/Psychology

Haridas Chaudhuri (1913–1975) was a psychologist. He had corresponded with Aurobindo and visited Aurobindo's ashram. He took up the mantle of developing integral psychology. Like Aurobindo, Chaudhuri used the term "integral" to include thinkers of the Indian renaissance and Western views, including those of the Gnostics and other spiritual perspectives (Herman 2018). In going beyond his predecessor, Chaudhuri argued for an integral psychology that was "open-ended, flexible, able to transform itself according to the demand of the fast-paced evolution of contemporary culture" (Herman 2018, 246).

For Chaudhuri ([1965] 2019), yoga is both psychology and art. It is a psychology to the extent that it is a science of the knowledge of the personality and the self in its totality. As an art it is "a way of achieving the total fulfillment of the self" (29). The self is understood to be multidimensional, including not only the conscious rational mind but also the unconscious and the superconscious. The superconscious aspect of the person is not objectively observable but is purely experiential. As such, introspection and self-observation are the appropriate methods to explore this aspect of the self. Chaudhuri emphasized that these methods are empirical in the original sense of the word. As we will see, the psychology, or the process of coming to understand the self, can be combined with the art to create a psychotherapy, or a method to achieve integration and dissolve the problems in living associated with psychopathology.

Chaudhuri ([1965] 2019) emphasized that the central goal of integral yoga/psychology is self-integration. Problems in living are the result of self-alienation. Emotional, social, and political suffering are all traceable to the buried discrepancies within. Elements of the personality, such as passion and reason, instinct and intellect, emotion and understanding, all vie for prominence and must be reconciled to overcome psychological suffering. Yoga is the path to bring these discrepancies—many of which are unconscious—into awareness so that they can be unified.

Chaudhuri ([1965] 2019) expressed agreement with the dynamic view of psychological functioning in that he saw the source of psychological problems to be conflict. Like Freud, he understood that conflict between unconscious contents and processes and the needs of the conscious mind was the source of suffering. For Chaudhuri, the unconscious is a limitless source of energy. The contents are not only the instincts but the archetypes and creative urges. The rational consciousness channels this energy to achieve socially supported goals. There are a number of ways one may attempt to resolve the inherent tension that exists between unconscious energy and the need to control this energy. For example, one may choose hedonism, perfectionism, or asceticism. All of these strategies ultimately fail because they elevate one aspect of the self and attempt to control others. The only solution that can provide lasting peace is integration. One must pay attention, come to terms with, and reconcile the unconscious processes and contents with the needs of the conscious rational aspect of mind.

These discrepancies or conflicting aspects of our psychology are at the root of all psychological suffering. This includes the experiences of depression and anxiety. Chaudhuri took these issues head on in his book *Mastering the Problems of Living* ([1968] 1975). Depression is often the result of failure, disappointment, disillusionment, and the imperfections all humans encounter. These experiences are not to be avoided; they are to be absorbed. Integration is achieved by metabolization of those experiences that cause sadness and despondency.

This also applies to anxiety. For Chaudhuri ([1965] 2019), "All mental disturbances, neurotic and psychotic, are ultimately traceable to anxiety….Many forms of abnormal behavior such as alcoholism, drug addiction, compulsive criminality, and juvenile delinquency are ultimately conditioned by anxiety" (53). Resistance is often at the core of anxiety—resistance to the inevitable flux of life as well as resistance to the feeling of anxiety. Ultimately, however, we must have the difficult feelings: "By accepting the anxiety of gradual self-development and creative freedom, one can transform anxiety into the energy of creative self-fulfillment" (Chaudhuri [1968] 1975, 67).

One aspect of Chaudhuri's work that is important in this context is his view of the self-as-individual. He saw each person as entirely unique, the result of distinctive experiences and encounters with other people in various cultures. He eschewed "rational psychological categories and typologies" (Shirazi 2018, 57). Additionally, "There is a unique path of development, growth and unfoldment for each individual which must be understood in terms of that person's unique *swabhava* [a unique set of qualities and characteristics] … Integral Psychology is sensitive to issues of individuality and the path of individual psychological growth and psychospiritual embodiment and evolution" (Shirazi 2018, 57).

Each person has a unique path of development, which suggests that theories of linear development in specific stages that culminate in a normative way of functioning (in most cases, this means functioning as Western upper-class white men do) cannot honor the individual. This openness to multiple ways of being is expanded beyond developmental theories to all systems of understanding the world: "Yoga calls upon man [*sic*] to rise above all theories and dogmas" (Chaudhuri [1965] 2019, 22). As we look at forms of Integral Psychotherapy, we will see that this ecumenicism includes an opening to different schools of therapy rather than allegiance to a single theoretical orientation.

This process cannot blinker the role of society in the creation of the self. Indeed, Chaudhuri's Integral psychology is fundamentally a relational psychology. The self is not an isolated individual: "There is no self-enclosed entity in the universe" (Chaudhuri [1965] 2019, 86).

The psyche cannot be fully integrated without realization of its relationship to nature, society, and indeed the cosmos. Psyche and cosmos are inseparable aspects of one concrete reality. The fundamental reality is neither the psyche nor the cosmos but the psyche-cosmos continuum. It is neither the isolated self nor the independent universe, but the self-in-the-universe or the universe-for-the-self.

From Aurobindo to Chaudhuri, we see the elaboration of a theory of the human mind as ideally a fully integrated phenomenon that recognizes and values all experience. Likewise, the human mind is a fully integrated part of the universe and shares this feature with all mindedness in the universe. This basic cosmology and psychology laid the groundwork for two related but different approaches to psychotherapy.

Integral Psychology/Psychotherapy

Several scholars and therapists have elaborated on integral philosophy and psychology and arrived at important ideas about how to engage in a holistic approach to therapy. Based on the work of Chaudhuri, two approaches to psychotherapy have been elaborated. Cortright (2007) represents one stream of Integral Therapy. Wilber (2000) represents a slightly different view on integral psychology, and from this work Forman (2010) has suggested an Integral Therapy that differs in important ways from Cortright's method.

Cortright

Cortright (2007) set forward a description of Integral Psychotherapy that represents a branch of the Aurobindo-Chaudhuri tree of integral psychology. He explained the term "integral" by indicating that Western and Eastern psychology (the latter rejected as spirituality in Western literature) both represent necessary but limited views of the human psyche. Within Western psychology, each school of therapy likewise focuses on limited but necessary aspects of human functioning. Eastern psychology is also divided into different perspectives that are all partially true.

According to Cortright's model, Western psychology represents the frontal or surface level of the psyche. There is a surface body, heart, and mind, explored by different systems of Western psychology. There are also the inner being, the true being, and the central being, which are the territory of Eastern psychology. The experience of true being is termed in Western thought as spiritual experience. The central being is the site of the "eternal core of the human psyche…our deepest psychological core and most authentic self" (Cortright 2007, 25). The inner work helps us integrate our highest authentic self; the outer work paves the way to be able to accomplish this. But if we fail to do the inner work, the outer work is not complete, for "when we ignore this authentic self, we drift far from our true path and experience alienation, fragmentation, and psychological pain" (27). In this statement, spiritual work is placed squarely as the province of psychotherapy. Within these levels and divisions, we see the need to integrate Eastern and Western thought along with different schools from both systems in order to address all of the various psychological needs people may bring to therapy.

Cortright (2007) echoed Aurobindo's epistemology as the way to study the human psyche: the outer dimensions or frontal self can be studied by objective observation that centers the five embodied senses. The inner dimension is best studied by "the most sensitive instrument known to psychology—human consciousness" (Cortright 2007, 26).

Having described his views concerning integral psychology, Cortright (2007) put forward some observations regarding Integral Psychotherapy. His version of the method is both a general framework or metatheory to organize therapy and a brand of psychotherapy. As a psychotherapy, it includes techniques from several different schools to achieve objectives. A given objective is based on the level of the psyche that is implicated. He maps a school of therapy onto each of the different levels of psyche. For example, if one is engaged in doing outer work aimed at external symptoms, one may employ cognitive and/or behavioral approaches to treatment. If one is working to eliminate deeper causes within, one will use techniques associated with psychoanalytic interventions. If therapy is targeting the lower emotional level, focused on instincts and impulses, one will employ more classical Freudian techniques. If one is working on the middle emotional level, more contemporary Relational psychoanalytic techniques may be more useful. For higher emotional levels, one will use more Jungian approaches (Cortright 2007). The ultimate goal is always the same: integration of the entire person on all levels.

Cortright's approach is not codified but dependent on the therapist's own integration. The integration of the therapist is considered to be a necessary prerequisite for this work. Indeed, the aspiration for awakening is foundational to becoming an integral psychotherapist. Between being fully present for the client and the integration of the therapist, treatment will unfold in the manner the individual client requires. This means that predetermined outcomes or goals in treatment are subordinated to the process itself. To accomplish this, the therapist proceeds by being open to divine guidance in the form of intuition. Cortright is clear that one should be ever mindful of the potential pitfalls of intuition (like mistaking counter transferential material for intuition). One must also center on emotions as important information, a basis for evaluation, a form of communication, and a means to direct behavior.

Wilber and Forman

Ken Wilber identified at one time as a transpersonal psychologist but relinquished that label. He now identifies as a philosopher. He based his version of integral psychology on the work of Sri Aurobindo but made his own significant additions and changes to the originating theory. He, like other integral theorists, advanced an ontology that is inclusive. He referred to the nature of reality as the "Great Chain of Being" (Wilber 2000). For Wilber, reality is composed of levels of existence, or levels of being and knowing. Each lower level is encased in a higher level, like Russian stacking dolls: "Each senior dimension transcends but includes its juniors, so that this is a conception of wholes within wholes within wholes indefinitely, reaching from dirt to Divine" (2000, 5).

Each level of existence is known in different ways (i.e., has its own epistemology). The innermost "doll" is matter, which is known by physics. Matter exists within life. Life is known through the discipline of biology. Next is mind, which can be known by psychology. He is clear that psychology is more than the materialist quantitative objectivist study of the mind that dominates in the West. The next higher level is soul, which can be known through theology. The third level is Spirit, the first cause, which is known by mysticism. From this perspective, different levels of being must be known by different procedures. Based on his understanding of the Great Chain of Being, he proposed a psychology that integrates science and spirituality.

Not only must science and spirituality be integrated, but Wilber also advocated that three dominant orientations toward consciousness are partial views of the phenomenon. For Wilber, behaviorism has reduced consciousness to that which can be observed by another. Psychoanalysts reduced consciousness to structures of the ego, and existentialism reduced consciousness to personal structures (Wilber 2000). Wilber set the task for himself to "honor and embrace every legitimate aspect of human consciousness" (2) as the goal of his integral psychology.

The integration of schools of therapy is based on the way that they all approach consciousness in the sense of awareness. Wilber stated that all major schools of therapy share the fundamental emphasis on heightening the client's awareness. He said, "The curative catalyst, in every case, is bringing awareness or consciousness to bear on an area of experience that is (or has been) denied, distorted, falsified, or ignored" (Wilber 2000, 99).

He also embarked on another integrative endeavor: to combine the structures—which he defined as stable patterns—of consciousness with the states of consciousness. The structures are the levels of the Great Chain of Being. There are also stable patterns or structures associated with various developmental lines. The states of consciousness are the natural and the altered states. The former includes the waking state, the dreaming state, the deep sleep state, etc. The latter include states achieved through the use of entheogenic drugs, meditation, near-death experiences, etc.

It is ultimately the lines or streams of development that distinguishes Wilber's integral psychology and later work by his students from Chaudhuri and Cortright's Integral Psychotherapy. The lines of development that receive attention in Wilber's integral psychology are those that have been empirically supported. A partial list includes : Morals, affects, self-identity, psychosexuality, cognition, ideas of the good, role taking, socio-emotional capacity, creativity, altruism, several lines that can be called "spiritual" (care, openness, concern, religious faith, meditative stages), joy, communicative competence, modes of space and time, death-seizure, needs, worldviews, logico-mathematical competence, kinesthetic skills, gender identity, and empathy" (Wilber 2000, 27).

He is clear that based on the findings of positivist research, these independent lines of development are normative: "Each developmental line itself tends to unfold in a sequential, monarchical fashion: higher stages in each line tend to build upon or incorporate the earlier stages, no stages can be skipped, and the stages emerge in an order that cannot be altered by environmental conditioning or social reinforcement" (Wilber 2000, 28–29).

For Wilber, problems in living are due in part to a failure to "grow up" (MacDonald and Friedman 2020). As we will see shortly, different therapeutic techniques are chosen on the basis of which developmental stage a person is in on a given line and what intervention is likely to help them move to the next stage.

Wilber synthesized his views of human psychology in his five-piece model called AQAL, with stands for all quadrants, all levels, all lines, all states, and all types (Marquis and Wilber 2008). Wilber is not a therapist. As noted, he identifies as a philosopher whose area of interest is the human mind. But his ideas concerning the nature of the mind have great implications for psychotherapy. Thus, it may not be surprising to learn that his theories have been taken up and applied to psychotherapy by his students. Among them is Mark Forman, who set forward his way of applying Wilber's AQAL system to treatment.

According to Forman (2010), "The major purpose of [Wilber's version of] an integral model…is to learn to use the insights of the various fields of human knowledge in a complementary way. Integral theory attempts to bring together the most possible multifaceted and effective solutions to individual and social problems" (10). Each discipline or field of study regarding humans blinkers an aspect of reality. Biologists see only the body. Psychologists may see only the individual. Sociologists can only see the communal. Forman calls for the integration of various disciplines in helping therapists learn about the human condition and how to aid people who are experiencing mental difficulties. This represents a far cry from restricting treatment to approaches that have been validated in randomized controlled trials or meta-analyses of said trials. Nonetheless, Foreman, as Wilber does, stays very close to the developmental theories that have been conducted in academic psychology settings.

Forman (2010) unpacked Wilber's AQAL model. For all quadrants, he explained that "Integral Psychotherapy accepts that the client's life can be seen legitimately from four major, overarching perspectives: subjective-individual, objective-individual, subjective-collective, and objective-collective. Case conceptualizations and interventions rooted in any of these four perspectives are legitimate and potentially useful in psychotherapy" (Forman 2010, 12).

Regarding stages, or levels of development, Forman (2010) observed that: "Integral Psychotherapy accepts that the identity development of the client will significantly impact the therapeutic encounter, including the shape and severity of the presenting problems, the complexity of the therapeutic dialogue, and the types of interventions that can be successfully employed. The identity development of the therapist also impacts his or her ability to empathize fully with the challenges of the client" (17).

For Forman, identity is "I" versus "not-I," or what many would call the sense of self. The integral model posits that the self or identity develops through three major phases (broken into subphases or stages):

1. Pre-personal or pre-egoic: The sense of self is fragile or not fully coalesced.
2. Personal or egoic: Self is primarily mental; personality and ego are fully formed.
3. Transpersonal or trans-egoic: The person no longer identifies primarily or exclusively with the ego.

There is one other form of identification that is a "non-level," which is non-dual realization or non-dual identification. It is not a stage of development proper. When one achieves this, all major dichotomies are seen as singular so that there is no differentiation between inner and outer, good and bad, etc. Note the difference here between this model and Psychosynthesis: for the latter, the higher Self is already and always there. In Forman's formulation, the higher self is a developmental achievement.

Forman (2010) suggested that the techniques associated with different schools of therapy are appropriate to different levels of identity development. From this integral perspective, "in the earlier stages of development a person will need greater external and concrete support (i.e., ego structure-building, behavioral interventions, etc.) and that a person in later stages of development will tend toward treatments that emphasize insight and reflection" (Forman 2010, 97).

While the stage of identity development is central to Forman's (2010) treatment process, as noted above, the AQAL model recognizes multiple areas of functioning where one's level of development is important: "Integral Psychotherapy accepts there are multiple lines or capacities in addition to self-system development. It expects that clients will be developmentally uneven and posits that different interventions aimed at different lines can be useful in therapy" (Forman 2010, 22). A person will move toward greater complexity and integration in relation to a number of areas of functioning. Self or identity development is, of course, one of those areas. A therapist should carefully assess where a client is situated in terms of the development of all those areas noted above by Wilber (2000), such as cognitive development, moral development, spirituality, etc.

Forman (2010) also discussed states of consciousness that are important considerations in treatment: "Integral Psychotherapy acknowledges the importance of temporary, altered states of consciousness, including psychopathological, regressive, and mystical states. Open discussion of altered states can be a major avenue of therapeutic dialogue, and the appropriate facilitation of positive altered states in therapy can provide the client with additional insight and healing" (24–5).

Wilber's AQAL model also includes types. Forman (2010) elaborated on types as "a wide variety of styles or types of knowing—according to gender, culture, and individual personality—and that are all equally valid" (27). Forman is looking here at behavior, motivation, and point of view. They represent "non-normative differences of epistemological style, not hierarchical difference of epistemological capacity" (27). This includes categories like the Meyers-Briggs taxonomy, the five factors of psychological understanding of personality, and the personality disorders as they appear in the *Diagnostic and Statistical Manual of Mental Disorders and the International Classification of Diseases.*

Integral Psychotherapy not only integrates different disciplines and cultural perspectives on the mind but also integrates a number of different theoretical approaches to treatment. This type of integration, which Wilber (2000) has referred to as unification, is justified on the basis on the all-encompassing ontology of integral psychology (Marquis et al. 2021). All perspectives represent different facets of a complex and comprehensive universe. Likewise, each person is a complex being. Different approaches to therapy are based on the developmental location of the individual. Forman (2010) has suggested that to cover these factors, a client can benefit from biological-pharmacologic interventions, Behavioral Therapy, Psychodynamic Therapy, Cognitive Therapy, Humanistic Therapy, Feminist Therapy, Multicultural Therapy, Existential Therapy, Somatic Psychotherapy, and Transpersonal therapies.

Conclusion

Integral philosophy/yoga is intimately concerned with the human mind. This created a clear path in creating an integral psychology, which was, in turn, translated into a few different forms of Integral Psychotherapy. While the method put forward by Wilber may be the more popularized form of Integral Psychotherapy, it differs in important ways from the theories of Chaudhuri and Cortright and the practice outlined by the latter.

The common threads between all of the thinkers noted here are based on the understanding that the universe is a highly complex singularity. In its complexity, there is no single system of thought or theoretical perspective that can encompass its totality. Therefore, in understanding and working with the human mind, there is a clear advantage to looking beyond Western psychology. Eastern psychology, as it appears particularly in yoga, must be honored. In addition, various other disciplines, like philosophy and study of religions, are important.

This multidisciplinary and multicultural view of the human mind leads the therapist to be free to select from a menu of therapeutic schools and different techniques and interventions. For Chaudhuri and Cortright, the choice is not based on outcome studies or meta-analyses but on the needs of the particular client. For Wilber and Forman, it is based on the client's location on grid of normative developmental lines.

The needs of particular clients can be understood by looking at a number of areas of functioning. And this represents a significant difference between Chaudhuri/Cortright and Wilber/Forman. For the former, we must understand how one's past affects their current functioning. How different experiences, including social context, have led the individual to function as they do today. For Wilber/Forman, there is a series of stages that everyone traverses. A particular client must be located in terms of their stage of development with the view of moving them to a normative higher level of functioning. In spite of these differences, the integrative approach to psychotherapy is aimed at helping clients integrate patterns and states of consciousness to achieve wholeness.

Holistic Practice Points

- The psychological and spiritual are not separate. Again, contemplate your understanding of these areas of human experience.
- There are multiple levels of consciousness that we work with to achieve well-being. Learn to help clients access these different levels. Learning ways to help clients enter altered states of consciousness like meditation, guided imagery, active imagination, shamanic journeying, hypnosis and self-hypnosis, and others is important.

- We are comprised of multiple parts or pieces that must be integrated to achieve well-being. As is the case in Psychosynthesis, unification and integration of the split self is key to well-being. Help clients value all of the aspects of their self rather than trying to help them eliminate parts that seem difficult.

- Intentionality plays a role in the healing process. Mindfully set your intention before you greet a client and throughout the intervention. The intention is always to help the client achieve their best life. Proximal intentions may be to understand what it's like to be this client, to consider how a client came to be as they are, or to deliver what the client needs most from you right now.

- A dispassionate attitude toward the contents of the unconscious is necessary to achieve well-being. Always register and acknowledge difficult reactions. A difficult reaction is a sign that points to the presence of unconscious material that must be made conscious and processed.

- Achieving the highest self is the ultimate goal of therapy, the royal road to well-being. This is more important than eliminating the symptoms of a diagnosis.

- For Cortright, the core cause of mental suffering is disunity. For Forman, the core cause of suffering is developmental delay. Learn multiple developmental models and assess how your client is functioning and why they may be functioning in that way. What purpose does it serve? What are the parts of themselves they have rejected? Why do they reject them? What do they need to integrate them?

- There is some disagreement about the nature of development in different versions of integral psychology. Chaudhuri and Cortright understand the need to honor the unique developmental process and needs of each client; Wilber has offered a detailed list of developmental lines with a clear progression for each line. Helping clients becomes the process of aiding them uncover or attain their highest self.

- Equally, there is divergence concerning the approach to treatment. For Cortright, it is not codified. Foreman's view is more highly structured. My view of holistic therapy (see chapter six) is clearly in keeping with Cortright.

- Multiple forms or schools or brands of therapy are useful and can be combined based on a unifying metatheory. For Foreman, the brand of therapy is dependent on the client's level of development. For Cortright, the form of therapy is based on the client's level of integration. In my research on therapist intuition (Stickle and Arnd-Caddigan 2019), therapists disclosed that they used their intuition to fit the brand of therapy to a client's needs in a given circumstance.

- The therapist's level of integration is a necessary prerequisite from Cortright's perspective. Do the work on yourself first.

Chapter Six

Mind-Centered Depth Therapy
Theoretical Foundations

I introduced a mind-centered depth approach to therapy in 2021. I discussed at length in that book a post-materialist metatheory on which this approach is based. This worldview provides a means of unifying different perspectives, disciplines, and schools of therapy. Thus, in keeping with Wilber's (2000) and Edge's (2011) requirement and consistent with Sri Aurobindo's (2001) integral psychology and Assagioli's ([1965] 2012) view, this holistic approach to therapy is unified by means of an overarching logic. We will briefly review how this metatheory supports the need to move beyond the medical model to help people heal.

There are several elements in my mind-centered depth approach that are common in other forms of holistic therapies: it is a psycho-spiritual-social-biological-energetic model. As is the case with Psychosynthesis and Integral Therapies, it is based on a view of the self as a central focus in treatment. However, we will see that the sense of self I posit is distinct from both prior treatment models. Also in keeping with Assagioli ([1965] 2012) and Aurobindo (Ghose 2001), the role of the more Freudian understanding of unconscious and the existence of unconscious phenomena that are beyond individual experience are recognized. A mind-centered depth approach also acknowledges the importance of emotions, not as the effect of neurochemical activity but as an expression of mind. In keeping with Thompson's (2019) understanding of spirituality as meaning-making, a mind-centered depth approach to therapy includes helping clients create or find meaning, which helps them identify direction and purpose for their lives. My mind-centered depth approach also finds a good deal of inspiration in a number of developmental models. More in keeping with Chaudhuri's ([1965] 2019) understanding of individual human mental functioning and distinct from Wilber's (2000) normative developmental perspective, mind-centered therapy looks at human mental functioning in terms of what may have been adaptive at one point but is no longer serving the individual. Finally, as I discussed in 2021, a mind-centered approach recognizes the importance of the body as a means of helping people reflect more easily on their minds.

In this chapter, I will discuss these theoretical elements of mind-centered depth therapy. In the next chapter, I will pull out various implications of this theory and discuss the practice of mind-centered depth oriented ways of doing therapy.

A Post-Materialist Model

One important aspect of a mind-centered approach is that it is a rejection of bio-reductionism and hence the medical model based on materialism. There are three aspects of the medical model of psychotherapy that are problematic from this perspective. First, the medical model is based on a materialist worldview: the belief that the brain and neurochemical processes create all experience. A mind-centered approach is unified by a post-materialist metatheory that posits that mind is real, fundamental, and ubiquitous (Arnd-Caddigan 2021). Second, the diagnostic categories that are central to the medical model do not adequately represent either the causes or the manifestations of people's mental suffering and thus hold a minor position in treatment objectives. Third, the approach to treatment based on the kind of evidence that is elevated in the evidence-based practice valued by the medial model has limited utility in helping a human being achieve mental wellness.

One of the most serious limitations of evidence-based practice is the belief that integrated approaches are illegitimate because they are not supported by outcome studies. But how could they be? Integrated approaches are typically created *ad hoc* in response to a client's needs. As we have seen, holistic approaches to psychotherapy see people as complex and each individual as unique. Therefore, differing perspectives on what contributes to well-being, what mitigates mental suffering, and what techniques a client is most likely to respond to must be considered and balanced. The mind-centered approach integrates not only several different theories of treatment but several different disciplines. All of the ways that humans have understood mind and mental well-being are potentially useful. This especially includes non-Western perspectives. In addition, in keeping with Assagioli's interests, the corpus of research on parapsychology is very important and helpful.

The Sense of Self

Sense of Self is a Fundamental Aspect of Mind

As we have seen, both Psychosynthesis and integral forms of therapy place a great premium on helping clients understand the self in order to achieve mental well-being. In *Intuition in Therapeutic Practice* (Arnd-Caddigan 2021), I stressed the need to focus on a client's sense of self when working from a mind-centered approach to therapy. As I have come more and more to see a mind-centered approach as fundamentally holistic, I continue to see working with the sense of self as a primary emphasis in therapy. The reason for this is because a sense of self is a fundamental aspect of mind and is more experience-near to most clients than the abstract concept of mind.

When I ask almost anyone, "Do you use the word 'myself'?" they say that they do. Almost everyone can relate to being a "self." Excepting people with severe psychopathology, we have the sense that we are individual subjectivities. The philosopher Galen Strawson (2017) made the point right off: we know exactly what subjects of experience are by simply being one. How do we know? It is fundamental: we all (with the possible exception of individuals with severe mental disorders) have a sense of being a mental presence. As Strawson (2017) put it, we *know* we are "a single mental thing that is a conscious subject of experience" (18).

From Strawson's (2017) perspective, there is experience, and there is the subject of experience (the title of his book). He defines self as the experiencer of experience. Experience is what it's like. What it is like to kiss somebody you're attracted to for the first time cannot be fully described as a set of biological processes. Experience requires an experiencer. The kiss must be experienced by somebody who is experienced as a self.

Can there be no sense of self? In a study I recently completed, a participant told me that they had a client who said he's not himself. He's not his original self. First off, this does not mean that he's not *a* self; he's just not the same self he was before. But even more basic is the question, when someone says "I'm not me," who is experiencing not being me? Who is making the comparison between what was me and what is now or that "I" am "someone else"? Who could observe and then say, "There is no me; I don't exist." Who is the "I" in that statement? So even when the sense of continuity of self is disrupted, there is still some self-ness operating in the deep background. Not being me is an experience. Who is the experiencer of that experience?

An experience (what it's like) is registered by the experiencer, but the latter is not simply a passive receiver. The experiencer is also an active agent. In some cases, the experiencer gates experience, allowing some qualia to enter awareness and disallowing others. In some cases, the experiencer registers the experience as if it were like a previously experienced event. All of this is to say that if we want to help people change their minds in order to bring about mental well-being, we work with their sense of self.

Multiple Selves and a Single Self

Self is fundamental to mind. But is there *a* self or many selves? Several thinkers discuss the multiple nature of selves. That is, self is not, in fact, singular (see, for example, Schwartz and Sweezy 2019). Strawson (2017) asked the question: who is experiencing themselves as multiple? There must be some self beyond the experience of multiplicity. In Strawson's (2017) words, "any explicitly self-conscious experience has to present as experience from one single mental point of view" (29). This point is supported by two thinkers who both look at the multiplicity of selves. Both Jung and Schwartz use the term capital *S* Self to designate some "over-self" that is the ground of the multiplicity of self. Psychosynthesis and Integral Psychotherapy are based on a worldview that there is one universal, holistic mind, and that this one mind is expressed as a multitude of separate, unique minds. And so it is with our experience of self. We experience ourselves as a singular, unitary entity. And yet we see that this singularity is expressed as multiple selves, or self states or parts.

When it comes to well-being, the question is the degree to which we are able to reflect on this multitude of patterns, as well as the degree to which we can experience them as integrated. Some self states are unwanted. And so we curtail the ability to reflect on them and own them. These are often called dissociated self states: we don't experience them as part of "me." We can't reflect on them. In mind-centered work, like the other holistic approaches to therapy, we help clients consciously experience multiple self states in order to integrate them into the Self. I find it helpful to look at the concept of self-states from three different vantage points: repeated patterns and individual experiences, the cultural contributions to one's sense of self, and the values that one experiences as a fundamental component of who they are.

Self: Personality, Identity, and Character

The variety of self-states is the amalgamation of both individual and social processes. I have found it helpful to use the heuristic of understanding a client's set of self-states in terms of three arenas: personality, identity, and character. These three concepts implicate both the individual and social contributions to the client's sense of self.

Personality

In common use, personality is thought of as a set of qualities that make each person unique. The variables in the set can vary just as much as the expression of those qualities. Consider the following: one person can be mean and smart and tidy. Another person can be nice and thrifty and considerate. We see here that there is only one variable they share (mean/nice) with different expressions. The other two are entirely different variables. This is an extremely simplistic example and only intended to make the following point: the number of different personalities that exist is nearly infinite. So in common usage, personality is the set of qualities that makes you different from everybody else.

Psychologists define personality as the expression of five basic traits: openness, conscientiousness, extroversion, agreeableness, and neuroticism. Openness includes the degree to which a person is eager to learn and experience new things. People high in openness also tend to be imaginative, creative, and insightful. Conscientiousness is one's ability to think things through while controlling impulses. Conscientious individuals can reflect on how their behavior is affecting others. They are organized as well as attentive to interpersonal connections. Extroversion is one's degree of comfort in large social gatherings. Extroverts like to be the center of attention. Most of us are familiar with the opposite of extroversion: introversion. These are not people who are socially awkward or anxious. They can socialize just fine. But they feel drained and need time alone to recharge after being around a lot of people. Agreeable people are altruistic: they really consider others. They are affectionate and highly prosocial. Neuroticism is one's degree of emotional instability, especially in the face of stress. A neurotic person often experiences mood swings and typically experiences high levels of anxiety and/or depression when under pressure.

Where does one's expression of these traits come from? Are we born with them? Do they come from inside us? Or are they the result of society and early interactions? The psychologists who study personality traits say both: nature and nurture. Environment and personal endowment. A little bit of genetics and a little bit of the way we were treated in early childhood.

Back in the old days, psychologists tended to believe that personality was fixed. When I started as a therapist, insurance companies wouldn't pay for treatment for personality disorders because they said that personality can't change. Since then, we've learned that it, in fact, does change as a matter of course. A study by Damien, Spengler, Sutu, and Roberts published in 2018 in the *Journal of Personality and Social Psychology* found that personality (as defined by ten specific traits, cumulatively assumed to measure thoughts, feelings, and behavior) is both stable and malleable. Most people showed change in one or more personality traits over the course of fifty years. Of course, individual differences varied widely, with some people showing marked change and others showing greater stability. The research was not designed to answer the question as to why personality changes or how to stimulate such change.

Enter the analysts. Psychoanalysts have always been centered on helping people change their personality. In fact, from a Psychoanalytic perspective, when we look at mental illnesses such as anxiety, depression, eating disorders, etc., the issue is not the diagnosis or the symptoms of the diagnosis. The symptoms and diagnoses are rather seen as the result of a person's way of perceiving and interpreting experience. The patterned ways in which one perceives and interprets experience is called their personality. A personality disorder is when the ways of perceiving and interpreting are overly rigid and can't be adjusted to fit appropriately to the context. The patterns tend to repeat, and the sense of self is in part the process of repetition.

In psychoanalytic theory, personality is rated on a spectrum from healthy to psychotic. The place on the scale represents the degree of flexibility in one's perceptions and interpretations. None of us can be located as a dot on the continuum. Rather, we move up and down a span on the line. Under optimal circumstances, when we're relatively unstressed, we are our healthiest and most flexible. Under stress, we tend to get more rigid. Healthy means that we can perceive a situation with openness, taking in and appreciating novel aspects and meanings. We interpret what is happening as something that may be familiar but is also different in subtle but important ways. The more newness in the way we perceive and interpret, the more we are able to learn and grow from new experiences. Of course, complete openness would mean that life would lose its predictability, and we would likewise have great difficulty functioning, let alone learning. So complete openness would not be healthy either.

When we become rigid, the *Psychodynamic Diagnostic Manual* (PDM Task Force 2006) indicates several areas where we tend to apply old experiences more rigidly. That is, we tend to see the world through a rigid set of central tensions or preoccupations. This is stuff like "life is harsh and unfair," we tend to fall back on rigid self states (like "I'm weak and incompetent"), we tend to see others as being just like important others from our past (other people want what they can get out of you), we tend to rely on a small set of defenses, and we tend to experience a small set of affective states. Lest these sound like cognitive distortions or cognitive schema, let me add immediately that these can function unconsciously. They can be feelings or physical reactions as well as fully formed thoughts.

The patterns that we look through have become endogenous, generated from inside a person, or based in part on one's unique, idiosyncratic processing of experiences. Two people can be in the same situation yet experience it very differently. Some of it may be based on things like intelligence, imaginative ability and play, and so on. Yet we must be aware of the importance of social environment in the creation of these patterns. Interpersonal interactions that occurred very early in life tend to be repeated over and over, even when they are no longer adaptive to the given environment. To go back to the relationship between experience and experiencer, personality is part of the experiencer that gates experience: the patterns let some experiences in and process them in a routine way and blocks other experiences. In mind-centered therapy, we look at the personality as a way to understand the patterns of perceiving and interpreting that gate experiences available to a client. We help clients expand the repertoire of what is possible while supporting a degree of predictability.

Identity

Sociologists look at identity and see it as a social construct. They stress that culture and interpersonal relationships shape how we experience ourselves as well as how others experience us. Identity is defined as "the set of meanings that define individuals as occupants of roles in society, members of groups or social categories, or unique persons with characteristics that identify them" (Burke and Stets 2023, 1). They are "internalized sets of meanings that can be found in culture that define who individuals are" (3).

Identity originates both endogenously (from within a person) and exogenously, or through processes between the individual and others (Burke and Stets 2023). I use the term "identity" in my work as a way of giving importance to exogenous influences on the sense of self. Roles and categories as well as the hierarchical valuing of different roles and placement in a category gives rise to power relations. Power relations, in turn, are a mechanism of oppression and marginalization or, in Thompson's (2019) words, alienation. When one group has the power to define the experiences of another group, this is oppression and leads the oppressed to be estranged from their authentic self or Self.

Identity theory is folded into a holistic approach to therapy in a few ways: helping the therapist determine what identities a client carries; understanding what those identities mean to them; and how well those identities fit or are integrated with an overall sense of self. Any of these three considerations may become a focus of change if they do not contribute to the client's wellness. Let's look at the example of gender. We are assigned a gender at birth based on our sex organs. Even before we are born, our parents may post a gender reveal on social media. They buy or are gifted toys and apparel that reflect girl or boy. As a child grows and interacts in the world, the designation "girl" or "boy" may be experienced as ego-syntonic, fitting with one's private experiences of themselves, or ego-dystonic, feeling strange, alien, or inaccurate. The degree to which private experience clashes or is consistent with social expectations and category and role assignment may be highly important to some clients' functioning. We may see ourselves as a different element in a social category than we are assigned (i.e., we may feel more like a girl even though we are socially seen and treated as a boy), or we may feel that we are completely outside of the category. We may feel that we are neither/both girl/boy or some entirely other designation. Again, in holistic therapy, it is important to understand what roles and categories a client has been placed into by others and how this relates to their subjective experiences of themselves and what the consequences are in terms of oppression, marginalization, and alienation.

When we talk about self, we must consider identity. We have to explore the way one relates to a cultural category they are placed in at birth. Is the category they were assigned considered inferior or superior? Does it adequately represent their subjective experience? Our purpose is to help our clients bring all of their experiences to a level of consciousness where they can elaborate, refine, and accept or reject social restrictions. The point is to help our clients feel like they can be authentic in their own skin. We therapists must be vigilant to assess how one's place in one or more categories is associated with oppression and marginalization and how oppression and marginalization create mental suffering.

Character

Once again, I use this term as a heuristic to help my clients reflect on different aspects of themselves. I use the term in keeping with ethicists to refer to moral qualities derived from values, which a person feels is a defining (at least aspirationally) aspect of their self. For example, I am a person who is trustworthy, or I am compassionate, or I am thrifty, etc. These qualities inform the way one thinks, acts, and feels. While character varies from person to person, it is also related to the social environment. This is so because our culture defines which character traits are valuable to a large degree.

I have found in my practice that individuals who cannot point to a set of virtues as part of their sense of self often experience life as flat or empty. I have come to see that having character, or the aspiration to embody certain virtues, is central to well-being. This is not to say that there are specific virtues that are necessary for well-being but to say that one must hold a set of aspirational characteristics—to be a person of character—to live well.

Of course, virtues can be held too rigidly, just like other ways of being in the world. We know that to always speak the truth can be a very bad idea. In some cases, being thrifty can be problematic. And so we hope to help our clients understand when and how to regulate the expression of their character.

The sense of self can be looked at as a combination of individual aspects and aspects that are culturally produced. The patterns of how one perceives and interprets experiences, the way they relate to the roles and categories that culture supports, and the values that they hold at their core are all going to have a profound effect on their well-being or suffering and form an important part of mind-centered treatment.

Consciousness and the Unconscious

Holistic therapies pay special attention to various levels or forms of consciousness. As we have seen in the preceding chapters, experiences in our awareness (conscious experiences) and experiences that we are not aware of or able to reflect on (unconscious experiences) are a central feature in holistic therapies. In Psychosynthesis, we saw that Assagioli ([1965] 2012) described a lower, middle, and higher unconscious. Sri Aurobindo (2001) described a lower unconscious and higher unconscious from which one can access a broader and higher range of experience.

The holistic approach to therapy that I am describing here is called a mind-centered depth approach because of the importance of unconscious processes and material in this type of treatment. It includes delving into the repressed unconscious, which can be aided by accessing altered states of consciousness. With some clients, it can include accessing higher states of consciousness and transpersonal insights, although it must be immediately noted that not every client wishes to engage in this level of treatment, and, of course, we never impose our values or ideas on them.

In the last few decades, some analysts have argued that while it remains central that we work with and change unconscious processes, it is not required that we make them conscious. The Boston Change Process Study Group (2010) has written extensively about "something more" than interpretation that drives change in therapy. This something more is change in unconscious/implicit processes, which are changed on the implicit level through the responsiveness of an attuned therapist. The Study Group has specified that implicit relational knowing is procedural knowledge of how to be with a specific other person. It is a "configuration of adaptive strategies that emerges" (5) from sequences of interaction in which each person in a dyad works to understand the other and the interaction in which they are engaged. When this process is successful, both parties are able to "integrate affect, cognition, and behavioral/interactive dimensions" (5), including unconscious material. This integration spurs both developmental and therapeutic aims when the therapist brings a greater degree of complexity, cohesiveness, and coherence to the interaction.

Members of the Boston Change Process Study Group, such as Tronick et al. (1999), have identified a similar process as dyadically expanded consciousness. This work suggests that the mind of one person, when connected to the mind of another in an intersubjective field, expands both minds or makes possible a greater area of awareness: one can reflect on and elaborate more and new experiences. Again, when one mind is more mature, in the case of development, or has greater complexity *in a specific area of experience* as in therapy, that complexity is shared with the client. The client now has a new degree of mental complexity, cohesiveness, and coherence in relation to specific experiences than previously. The Study Group identified the "sloppy process" of searching for, finding, losing, and refinding the client. This process is mutative in that it helps the client integrate nonconscious material. Connecting to another mind expands our consciousness. This may be very close to the Psychosynthesis notion of "spontaneous irradiation" (Nocelli 2021, 92) in which minds directly influence each other. Expansion of consciousness includes both helping clients reflect on a larger portion of their experiences as well as experiencing in new ways that have hitherto been outside of their repertoire. This expansion is an important aspect of a mind-centered holistic approach to psychotherapy.

Emotions

Thompson (2019, 2020, 64-71) stressed that emotions must return to the center of psychotherapy. Just exactly what an emotion is may be as disputed as what consciousness is. There are several neurochemical explanations of what emotions are and where they come from (see, for example, Damasio 1994). There are also several cognitive theories of emotions (for example, Ellis 1962). Both of these approaches to emotions suggest that they are epiphenomena of other, more fundamental processes. If an approach to psychotherapy is to be truly holistic, we refrain from reductionism and thus do not try to relieve negative feelings by manipulating the body or altering thoughts that are secondary to the feelings. We deal with the feeling qua feeling. We do not try to extinguish emotions but rather integrate and use feelings as vital information.

Emotional intelligence is a construct that has received a great deal of attention since the 1990s. There is a body of research that supports the notion that the ability to identify emotions, regulate emotions, use information that emotions contain, and integrate emotions into thought are capacities that are related to mental well-being (see, for example, Extremera and Fernandez-Berrocal 2006). Emotional intelligence is an important component in a mind-centered approach to therapy.

Emotion is a construct that intersects with several components of holistic psychotherapy, including meaning-making, the sense of self, and the unconscious. The ability to create/assign meaning is an important element in holistic therapy. But where does meaning reside? According to the Boston Change Process Study Group (2010), affect is at the very center of meaning-making. Affect gives experience valence, and the affective valuation of experience is the primary source of meaning. Greenberg (2004) has supported this observation: by imparting this information, emotions contribute to meaning.

Emotions are also at the core of the sense of self. Fonagy et al. (2005), together and individually (see, for example, Jurist 2019), have explored the relationship between affect and the sense of self at length. I discussed the view of the development of the self from the perspective of analysts and developmental psychologists in a previous publication (Arnd-Caddigan 2021). In a nutshell, our caregivers must reflect us to us in order for us to develop a healthy, realistic sense of self. Much of this reflection occurs when they match our vitality affect (our emotional state and the intensity of it) when we feel good and can regulate us when we feel bad. That is, they must accurately judge our feeling state and respond appropriately by sharing or changing that state. If a caregiver cannot determine our state but is instead overwhelmed by their own emotions, we begin to develop what Fonagy et al. (2005) has called an "alien self." Thus, the interplay of two people in relation to an emotional state plays a large role in the sense of self.

Unconscious emotions have been the cornerstone of Psychoanalytic Psychotherapy since Freud (2004). But for those who are not analytically trained, the concept may at first appear to be an oxymoron:

unconscious emotions are "feelings that are not felt" (Winkielman and Berridge 2004). Historically, there has been widespread belief among many psychologists that attention can bring emotion into full awareness and/or that the very definition of emotion requires awareness (Winkielman and Berridge 2004).

However, this appears to not be the case. Research supports Freud's original understanding that unconscious emotions can drive behavior and physiological reactions (Winkielman and Berridge 2004). Implicit emotions create changes in "experience, thought, or action" (Winkielman and Burridge 2004, 121). As the authors observed, given that emotions are important information about our environment, the ability to use that information to react does not require conscious reflection. Indeed, the time and effort that reflection requires may be a hindrance to a speedy reaction.

Jurist (2018) also noted that emotions can be unconscious. He stated at the very outset of his book that "Acknowledging that we do not fully know what we feel is crucial....The experience of not knowing our feelings is an everyday part of our lives" (1). He termed those emotions that we cannot explicitly identify as "aporetic emotions," which he defined as those emotions that are difficult to know. In Jurist's (2018) view, bringing those "obscure, mystifying, or confusing mental states" (1) into conscious awareness to the degree possible (it is not completely possible) is necessary for identifying, modulating, and expressing emotions. These capacities are bedrock to self-understanding and understanding others and therefore psychological well-being.

Not only is it possible for emotions to be unconscious, but emotions are key to the unconscious. In my clinical experience, it is often the case that strong emotions erupt from clients when unconscious material is close to breaking into awareness. If we stay with the feeling, we can move toward a great deal of repressed content. We avoid lapsing into intellectualization to collude with the client's defenses.

We see then that in holistic therapy, we work directly with emotions with the objective of helping our clients to recognize, tolerate, modulate, and integrate a full array of emotions. There was a time when therapists thought that helping clients reduce certain difficult emotions was helpful (Jurist 2018). But in fact, all emotions are important and must be given a central place in therapy. We help our clients become aware of the emotions that are working on an unconscious level and how this affects their way of being in the world. We teach our clients to mine adaptive information from emotions and modulate (without eliminating) them when they are overwhelming.

One aspect of emotions that is particularly important in mind-centered therapy is the emotions of the therapist as they arise in a session. These are not mere distractions that must be sequestered. Your emotions during a session are very important information. Is this a feeling that you have had with other clients, other people in your life? If the answer is yes, then it may be something that is emerging from your unconscious that can inform you about your own stuck patterns of being with certain other people. It may be a sign that you are missing something important about the client's experience because you are filtering it through your own. But if the answer is no, then this may represent important information about your client.

To take a single example, I had a patient who evoked in me a whole gamut of unpleasant feelings. It would have been very foolish of me to ignore these feelings or consider them my own neurotic reactions since this patient's principal complaint was her terrible unpopularity. The way she affected me was a function of her psychopathology—a function of utmost importance to her and one that it is crucial for us to understand (Segal 1992, 14).

In other words, feelings that arise in you during therapy may be a window into how your client feels or how others routinely feel about or around your client.

Long ago, the analyst Racker (1957) noted that countertransference can take two forms: complimentary and concordant. Racker identified concordant countertransference to be a form of empathy. That is, the therapist is feeling what the client is feeling. Today, we see this as a form of unconscious communication: the therapist "contages" the client's often unconscious feelings. If the therapist is able to maintain the bifocal awareness on their clients and on their own internal/emotional state on a moment-to-moment basis, the therapist may be able to use the emotions that arise in them and, in some cases, ask the client if the feeling seems familiar. In other cases, the feeling the therapist can discern may be complimentary countertransference. Complimentary countertransference is represented as feelings in the therapist that the client evokes. They may be reactions the client likewise evokes in others. The questions become, "Is this what it's like for most people to be with this client? Does the client live surrounded by people who feel like this around them? What might this client experience if others frequently feel this way around them? How might this influence the client's sense of self?"

We see then that the therapist's emotions are important in therapy and the client's emotions—both conscious but especially their unconscious emotions—are a central area of focus in a mind-centered depth approach to therapy.

Systems of Meaning-Making

The meaning that experience has for clients is a key feature of a mind-centered approach to psychotherapy. A very long time ago, I cited Lakoff (1988) and Nelson (1985) in observing that meaning is elaborated on three levels: the individual, the interpersonal, and the cultural. Individuals differ in the way that they elaborate meaning. For example, one's capacity for abstractions, their ability to reflect, and their imaginative capacity will influence what a given event will mean to them. Much meaning is communicated interpersonally, especially in the family. Our parents and siblings share their meaning with us as if it were truth, and we often adopt that meaning without question. Of course, our culture transmits a great deal of meaning, often through the medium of categories. There is another level of meaning I would add at this point: the transpersonal. We have the capacity through altered states of consciousness to acquire new meaning that we have not encountered on the other three levels.

Perhaps one of the most identifiable aspects of holistic psychotherapy is the acknowledgment of the relationship between spirituality and psychotherapy. Both of these phenomena are foundational to the way that clients make meaningful lives. We must immediately acknowledge that not all clients are interested in spirituality or religion. I have found that in most cases, these people lean heavily toward one or another philosophical school, even if they are not aware that such a school of philosophy exists. Thus, along with Thompson (2019, 2020, 64-71), I believe that we should expand the notion of religion and spirituality to include philosophies or any system of meaning-making that our clients can draw on to help them live a higher quality of life.

As much as there appears to be more interest in the intersection between psychotherapy and religion/spirituality, therapists continue to receive inadequate training in this area. For example, Vogel et al. (2013) conducted a study of training in religion and spirituality in psychology programs and found that there were several lacuna in training overseen by the American Psychological Association. Moffatt et al. (2021) found that only about one-third of master of social work programs have explicit courses that address religion/spirituality. This was somewhat offset by the fact that this material is being increasingly incorporated across the curriculum. Audate (2022) has noted that many practitioners feel ill prepared to explore religion and spirituality in their clinical work. This comes up frequently in my supervision with associate-level licensees. The early-career therapists hear their clients alluding to religion and/or spiritual interests or concerns but are uncomfortable pursuing the topic. They feel that engaging clients in this domain is malpractice. I am unclear where these therapists have gotten this idea, but it is a repeated theme in supervision. As we examine the role of spirituality in holistic approaches to psychotherapy and counseling, we must be mindful of the need to provide adequate training in how to accomplish this.

Vieten and Scammell (2015) have set forth competencies for working with clients around the issues of spirituality and religion for psychotherapists and mental health professionals. They have stressed that our clients are spiritual or religious and want to talk about issues around their spirituality and/or religion in therapy. Even when a client does not present with a specifically spiritual or religious concern, their beliefs and practices are important to their overall psychological functioning in both positive and negative ways. We must be able to help clients call upon strengths that spirituality and religion confer as well as help clients come to terms with ways their spirituality or religion may be causing harm.

While the research is consistent that religion and spirituality can confer psycho-social benefits to those who engage in related beliefs and practices, we must also be mindful of spiritual abuse and religious trauma and be prepared to work with our clients around these issues. Religious trauma results from an event, series of events, relationships, or circumstances within or connected to religious beliefs, practices, or structures that is experienced by an individual as overwhelming or disruptive and has lasting adverse effects on a person's physical, mental, social, emotional, or spiritual well-being.

Religious trauma is widespread:
After compiling data from 1,581 adults living in the United States, this study concludes it is likely that around one-third (27–33%) of U.S. adults (conservatively) have experienced religious trauma at some point in their life. That number increases to 37% if those suffering from any three of the six major RT symptoms are included. It is also likely that around 10–15 % of U.S. adults currently suffer from religious trauma if only the most conservative numbers are highlighted. Nonetheless, since 37 % of the respondents personally know people who potentially suffer from RT, and 90 % of those respondents know between one and ten people who likely suffer from RT, then it could be argued that as many as one in five (20 %) U.S. adults presently suffer from major religious trauma symptoms (Slade et al. 2023, 1).

We must be ready and able to address the meaning system the client was socialized into early in life. Then we must inspect how that meaning system impacts the client today. We must understand the way they create meaning and how this operates on conscious and unconscious levels to create both resiliency and harm.

Developmental Models

We have seen that there appears to be some disagreement among integral therapists on the role of developmental theories in a holistic approach to therapy. Chaudhuri ([1968] 1975) appears to champion the view that the normative nature of these theories blinkers the uniqueness of each individual experience. Wilber (2000) is clear that his psychology includes emphasis on several developmental models as important indices of where change should be targeted.

As Thompson (2020, 64-71) noted, a truly holistic approach to therapy must include the social aspects that contribute to individual functioning. People develop in response to their physical and social environment. This is perhaps the most important observation of the extensive literature on attachment theory. We thus want to understand how a person is functioning in any developmental area and whether it is currently adaptive. Being aware of several different developmental theories is helpful, but there is no single list of developmental accomplishments that is final. The question is not ultimately which developmental theory I think is important and how I think the client should be functioning in that area but rather how this person is functioning that is contributing to their problems in living. How could they change to achieve greater well-being? A developmental theory may give us some insight but does not dictate the a priori goal for treatment. Some theories of human functioning that are often described in terms of development that I find to be helpful are personal epistemology, emotional and social intelligence, mentalization, and morality, though this is by no means intended to be a prescriptive or exhaustive list.

The Body

The biological aspects of self have been at the very center of the discipline of psychology since its inception. We have seen that many approaches to holistic therapy include a host of somatic interventions. In any form of therapy the unity of body-mind is important to always keep front of mind. However, in our culture we have lost touch with our minds to a large extent. We see our bodies as ourselves. A mind-centered approach attempts to help clients experience their bodies, thus awakening them to their minds/selves. For example, in my work, I use a variation of Emerson's (2015) approach to yoga. But rather than using this approach with the idea that the body movement somehow unlocks some distress that resides in the body, I use the approach to help my client become aware of their mind/self. I use yoga to help clients open to the experience of their bodies and help them recognize themselves as experiencers of physicality. This is a very different emphasis. Thus, while mind-centered psychotherapy does not blinker the body, we attempt to balance a person's acknowledgment of themselves as much more than their bodies.

Conclusion

The mind-centered approach to holistic psychotherapy, like other forms of holistic therapy, offers a viable alternative to the medical model by looking at people as more than categories of illness and providing treatment that is not based on the logic of evidence-based practice. From this perspective, the self is fundamental to mind, and therefore, if we want to help our clients change the ways they experience the world, we work to help them open their sense of self. While there are multiple self states that are optimally integrated, helping clients to become aware of a central organizing self can bring them enhanced well-being. To accomplish this, I use the heuristic of seeing issues of personality, identity, and character. These three ways of looking at a person can help us understand how their personal endowments and experiences as well as the culture and interpersonal contexts in which they developed have come together to bring them a sense of who they are and who they wish to be. We also look at the unconscious and the conscious, and in keeping with other depth psychologies, we help our clients bring more and more experience into awareness. Likewise, we work with our clients' emotions directly. We look at their system of meaning-making to help them live with direction and purpose. Finally, we look to see how the environment has shaped their development, in some cases helping them to change their mental functioning.

Holistic Practice Points

- A mind-centered approach to holistic therapy is an alternative to the medical model. Avoid the temptation to overfocus on symptoms and diagnoses. Instead, stay centered on asking yourself how this client experiences their life and what they need most to experience it in more rewarding ways.
- The approach is based on the notion that mind and self are two aspects of a single phenomenon. If we wish to help our clients change the way they experience life (i.e., their minds), we help them by changing their sense of self. Explore all the aspects of your clients' sense of self and how they developed. Look closely for those aspects of self that are unconscious and how they leak into your client's functioning in disruptive ways.
- While there are multiple self states, there is ultimately a singular mental point of view. Ultimately, this singular self is integrated. Help clients know their "parts" and appreciate the self as an expression of something higher.

- The self can be understood as having three characteristics: the patterns of ways we experience, the roles and categories our culture places us in, and those virtues we hold as deep expressions of our self. Exploring all of these aspects of self is important in therapy.

- The self has important aspects that we can reflect on and important aspects that operate outside of our awareness. Well-being is associated with enlarging the areas of awareness. Help clients do so by coming to awareness through conversation, interpretation, and altered state of consciousness techniques.

- Emotions are important to our sense of self and the ways that we elaborate meaning. They are a central focus in a mind-centered approach to therapy. Help clients become aware of unconscious emotions and stay with difficult emotions. The ability to learn from and integrate them is crucial to wellness.

- Having meaning, purpose, and direction are central to well-being. Clients can call on philosophy, religion, and/or spirituality to help them live a meaningful life. We must also be aware that some systems of meaning-making can cause great harm. Discussing spirituality and opening the conversation to explore potential spiritual abuse is important.

- Developmental theories identify very important aspects of human mental functioning. Knowing a multitude of such theories can help us understand how our clients experience their lives. We must be careful to note that optimal functioning in any of these areas is contextualized by the social environment. Do not infantilize your client by assuming that they are regressed or delayed. Instead, look for the protective function of their current state of development.

Chapter Seven

Mind-Centered Depth Therapy Practice Considerations

We have looked at several theoretical aspects of a mind-centered approach to holistic therapy. These features can be linked to objectives for treatment. We help our clients integrate multiple self states into a unified self. We guide them as they develop a more flexible personality. We help them to understand how social forces impact their identity in order to mitigate the effects of oppression and marginalization. We help our clients develop their character. We guide our clients as they integrate the personal unconscious and perhaps experience Superconscious. Our clients benefit from an increased ability to identify, integrate, and modulate a full range of emotions. We help our clients develop meaning, direction, and purpose, frequently in the context of religious, spiritual, or philosophical systems. We help our clients understand how their past experiences affect them, taking into consideration how functioning in several developmental areas may be hampering their efforts at well-being. We also help our clients connect to an experience of their bodies, using their concrete embodiment to help them embrace their minds.

How do we do this? The answer does not lie in techniques. Rather, the mind-centered approach to holistic therapy is a reflective practice. The practitioner must be able to use the common factors that underly all effective forms of therapy. With those basics, from a mind-centered depth perspective, connection, intention, and attention are the means of determining exactly how we can help our clients change.

Reflective Practice

A mind-centered approach to therapy is not dependent on techniques. How we approach our clients from this perspective is not manualized. We may decide to use techniques that other therapists have shared with us, that were developed in spiritual contexts (like meditation or shamanic journeying), or that are published as methods used in specific brands of therapy (like Socratic questioning or tapping). What determines which technique we use (or if our only technique is to engage in a conversation) is decided by what our client can use for their healing. Put differently, a mind-centered depth approach to psychotherapy is a reflective practice as opposed to a technical-rational practice.

Schon (1984) long ago discussed the rise of technical-rationality, problems with this approach for professional practice, and an alternative approach that he termed "reflection-in-practice." According to Schon (1984), technical-rational practice is applied science that "yields diagnostic and problem-solving techniques which are applied in turn to the delivery of services" (24). The services are targeted to achieve clearly defined specified and circumscribed ends. That is, it is the application of specific techniques to accomplish predetermined bite-sized goals. Manualized treatment protocols and the prescribing of specific techniques for specific diagnoses or symptoms are examples of technical-rational practice. As Schon (1984) observed regarding technical-rational practice, "the researcher's role is distinct from, and usually considered superior to, the role of the practitioner" (26).

The ideal of technical-rationality cannot provide an adequate response to problems that are complex, in a context of uncertainty and instability, in a situation with unique or unpredictable elements, or where there are value conflicts regarding the appropriate goal (Schon

1983). Schon himself used mental health as an exemplary of a profession in which these circumstances dominate. He separated psychotherapists into two groups: those who distinguish "patients as examples of standard diagnostic categories" and those who see the patient as a "unique case...a universe of one" (Schon 1983, 108). These latter practitioners engage in reflection-in-action: "Knowing is ordinarily tacit, implicit in our patterns of action and in our feel for the stuff with which we are dealing...in his day-to-day practice he makes innumerable judgments of quality for which he cannot state adequate criteria, and he displays skills for which he cannot state the rules and procedures. Even when he makes conscious use of research-based theories and techniques, he is dependent on tacit recognitions, judgments, and skillful performances" (Schon 1983, 49–50).

Yet even while the reflective practitioner seems to be acting automatically, they "think about what they are doing, sometimes even while doing it...they turn thought back on action and on the knowing which is implicit in action....As he tries to make sense of it, he also reflects on the understanding which have been implicit in his action, understanding which he surfaces, criticizes, restructures, and embodies in further action" (Schon 1983, 50).

From Schon's perspective, a good psychotherapist is like a good jazz musician. As the musicians listen to themselves and each other, they are able to make adjustments on the spot, albeit psychotherapists act within the parameters of a psychotherapeutic session.

This kind of practice requires a very wide-ranging theoretical knowledge and practice (as well as life) experience: it requires both knowledge and wisdom. While the stereotype of a holistic therapist may be that of someone who is ungrounded and unprofessional, in fact, holistic therapists are committed, knowledgeable professionals. It may be because of the extraordinary knowledge and experience base required to do this kind of work that insurance companies and certain mental health agencies require technical-rational practice. However, with appropriate training and supervision, a new clinician is able to rise to this level of practice ability.

Connection, Intention, Attention

If techniques are not the most important mutative factor in holistic therapy, we need to be clear on what it is that we do that promotes healing in our clients. From a mind-centered depth perspective, we find that the connection between the therapist and client is the factor that guides the process. We have learned from research on energy and indigenous healers that the intention the healer sets is a crucial aspect of the process. This combination of the connection and healing intention allows us to trust the path carved by our attention. Our attention is informed by intuition, formal theory, and past experience.

Connection (Fittedness)

From a holistic perspective, we have a wealth of techniques and exercises we can introduce to clients. We can use various systems of intentional movement (yoga, dance, qigong, etc.); we can use manipulation of the body (tapping, etc.); we can use any of the myriad forms of meditation (mindfulness, guided meditations, active imagination, etc.); we can use any of the creative arts, and on and on. But these tools are not the primary mutative factor from a mind-centered perspective. They can be very helpful, but they can also be a distraction or empty exercises. More important than techniques is the connection, or fittedness, between the therapist and client.

The members of the Boston Change Process Study Group (2010) have highlighted the degree to which the specific techniques we use are not the principle means of triggering change with clients. They have shown that the quality of the intervention is not a matter of "theoretical or technical proficiency on the part of the therapist" (Boston Change 2010, 199). Rather, the quality that matters is that of the relationship. Relational quality "has to do with how well an act or statement [or the use of a technique] on the part of the therapist or patient advances the directional fittedness and expands the shared relational field between them" (Boston Change 2010, 199). In this relational field, the minds of both the client and the therapist are expanded to allow new experiences to emerge; a new sense of self to begin to take shape.

Stern (2017) has discussed a related concept. He recommended that the therapist center on this question: What does this client need from me? If a technique fits with the client's (often unconscious) need, it will move the process forward. The movement toward health is advanced by the increased fittedness in the relationship. That is, the therapist's ability to know what the client needs and if and/or which technique may be helpful is a result of enhanced Fittedness.

Fittedness is augmented by the twin operations of attunement and regulation. Stern (1985, 77–92) observed caregivers attuning to infants very early in life. This is the process of matching another's vitality affect. Vitality affect is the intensity (vitality) and emotion (affect) of another. Stern stressed that this is often accomplished cross-modally. In other words, an infant may be moving their arms and kicking their legs with excitement, and the caregiver will vocalize with the same intensity and rhythm as well as the same degree of excitement. I see students in mock interviews in class frequently nodding their heads as their partner speaks, nodding with the same intensity and at the same rhythm as the speaker's vocalizations.

Attunement is a great way of connecting to others when they are in an ego-syntonic state, that is, when they feel in a comfortable state for them (people are comfortable with different levels of feeling and stimulation). When an infant is in an ego-dystonic state (under- or overstimulated, unhappy/uncomfortable, etc.), the caregiver regulates them by adopting a vitality affect that is closer to the infant's optimal range. So when an infant is understimulated, the caregiver will shake a rattle quickly with a high voice and rapid vocalizations. When the infant is overstimulated, the caregiver will relax their muscles and rock the baby slowly and gently with a slow, low, quiet voice. When we engage in this behavior with a client, not only does it help them learn to regulate their own feelings, but they realize that another is connected to their pain and able to help them out of it. This is a good example of how connection requires fittedness: we must be able to discern what the client needs at this moment.

Because minds can connect, the most important mutative factor in mind-centered therapy is the connection between the mind of the therapist and client. This concept has been alluded to in much psychoanalytic theory. Human minds have the ability to share subjectivity or combine to create intersubjective experiences (Stern 1985, 77–92). It is this connection that drives all of the choices a mind-centered clinician makes. As is the case in Person-Centered Therapy (Rogers 1957), the connection between the client and therapist is not just a necessary condition for treatment but is a mutative factor in treatment.

How do you do that? First and foremost, you have to be secure enough in your own sense of self to allow yourself to open to another. All connections are two-way. A few psychoanalytic practitioners have discussed the degree to which a client can come to know about their therapist due to the bidirectional nature of unconscious communication (Bass 2015). You must have done your own work. You must have a degree of security, centeredness, and self-awareness.

This third factor is especially important because, as discussed in *Intuition in Therapeutic Practice* (2021), it is easy to confuse what is yours and what is coming from your client during unconscious communication. Knowledge of your own patterns of perception and interpretation of interpersonal experiences will go a long way in helping you discern which is which. Equally important is the ability to acknowledge when the client knows something about you that you did not intend to share, then gently turn the focus back to their minds.

The second step is to earn permission from your client to connect on this level. You cannot connect with someone who does not want to do so. Your client may reasonably or unreasonably fear intrusion, manipulation, judgment, or any one of number of bad intentions. They may have experienced painful connections in the past. Therefore, you must build trust with your client and earn their assent in engaging in this mentally intimate experience. The "therapy before the therapy" may be earning trust and gaining your client's permission to form a connection.

In my research on intuition in psychotherapy (Stickle and Arnd-Caddigan 2019), I learned that some therapists practice a small exercise to establish a connection with their clients. They reported visualizing a connector, like a bridge or a beam of light, between themselves and their client. Some people are not very visual, so imagining a sound that envelopes you both, a vibration between the two of you, or any other kind of imaginary experience might prove helpful. Like riding a bike, you need to find what works for you but mostly what works for your client.

Intention

Intention is an important element in energy healing, including Reiki, noncontact Therapeutic Healing, and a host of indigenous healing methods (Zahourek 2020). Zahourek (2020) has suggested that intentionality is the matrix of healing. There are a number of studies that support this contention. Beyond the general efficacy of intention in healing, there are a number of psychoanalytic thinkers who have stressed the importance of intention in psychotherapy. Taken together, we see that setting your intention is an important aspect of a mind-centered approach to therapy.

There are a number of studies that support the notion that intention can have a concrete impact on an identified target. Both the research on distant mental influence on living systems (DMILS) and distant healing intention (DHI) have supported the idea that one's intentions can have an effect on another living system. An important aspect of this research is the definition of intention that the researchers have developed. Schlitz et al. (2003) proposed definitions and guidelines for research on DHI. They defined DHI as situations in which "the intentions of one or more persons can interact with the physiological, psychological, and/or behavioral status of one or more distant living systems" (Schlitz et al. 2003, 31). Furthermore, an intentional action requires that the healer "1. Had a desire for an outcome; 2.

Had a belief that the action would lead to that outcome; 3. A desire to actually perform the action; 4. The skill to perform the action; and 5. Awareness of fulfilling the intention while performing the action" (32). This last point is important; the holistic therapist who uses intentionality as a means to aid healing for a client must carry out some action that is "a conscious and willful action" (Schlitz et al. 2003, 32). Thus, I am suggesting that we must do more than hold an intention for healing for our clients. We must engage in a practice—use a technique or engage in a conversation/dialogue, such as intuitive inquiry (Arnd-Caddigan 2021) with the explicit intention of promoting healing for our clients.

Intention defined in this way has been shown to be an effective means of promoting changes in living systems, including as a means of promoting healing. From 1977 to 1991, William Braud conducted a series of experiments with his associate Marily Schlitz on DMILS. The research methods included "directed intentional effort of a person to change a defined variable of a remote living system and the fluctuation of that variable" (Schmidt 2015, 244). Meta-analyses of the DMILS studies indicated that setting an intention to influence another system at a distance created the intended changes in those systems. In the same vein, Shiah et al. (2022) have demonstrated that Buddhist monks directing the intention to promote growth were able to do so in mesenchymal stem cells.

Likewise, Schlitz et al. (2003) have reviewed several studies on the effect of intentions on the physiological processes of animals and humans. In several related studies, there have been consistent findings that the influencer can intentionally evoke a response in another, even when a number of controls have been implemented and there is no direct contact between the influencer and the influenced.

Psychoanalytic thinkers have equally stressed the role of intentions in psychological healing. The Boston Change Study Group (2010) has discussed intention and its role in the co-creation of meaning in interaction. These authors observed that the ability to determine another's intentions is a basic human capacity. They concluded that when two people are involved in conversation, they can know what the other person's intentions are for the conversation. What this means is that if you sit with a client and are holding the intention to place them in the correct diagnostic category or to suss out what exactly is wrong with them, there is a good chance that your client will have a subtle unconscious reaction to your efforts. This may trigger an already poor self-concept or a shame response; it may trigger defensiveness or resistance. There are any number of appropriate responses to an intention to find and/or fix the pathology in a client. I am proposing that most of them are not healing.

Grossman (2023) has discussed the intentions of the analyst in the treatment process. While he stressed the role of attitude, he alluded to a key intention: the intention to "relieve suffering via the expansion of understanding" (115). From this perspective, intentionality for healing follows the lead of alternative forms of healing across cultures. For Grossman (2023), the intention to promote healing is accompanied by two important attitudes: to put the client's needs before those of the therapist and to hold deep respect for the client's suffering.

Given the power of intention, it is a good practice to be explicit about one's intention. The intention in a mind-centered approach to psychotherapy begins with two aims: to center on understanding another human being and to understand what they need from you to contribute to their growth (Stern 2017). Spoiler alert: part of what they need may be to help them engage their curiosity and creativity regarding mind—their mind, other peoples' minds, and Mind beyond.

Attention

Once you have established a connection and set a healing intention, the third feature of a mind-centered approach to psychotherapy is attention. On what do you train your attention? What pulls your attention in one direction or another? I have found there to be three sources of knowledge that draw clinicians to explore one aspect of what the client has just said versus another: intuition, formal theory, and past clinical experience. In *Intuition in Therapeutic Practice*, I discussed intuition at length, and intuition is one of the main triggers for what we respond to in relation to our client. Something the client just said feels important, or stands out in some way. For me, when my client is speaking sometimes certain words or phrases feel hot. Honing your intuition and learning to discern intuition from your own needs is important.

As a holistic approach, there are an almost infinite number of theories that can help give us insight into how this person is functioning and how they might alter their functioning to feel better. Psychological theories of development can provide an important window into specific areas of functioning that may be contributing to our client's mental suffering. In addition to all of the areas of development identified by the integral therapists, psychological theories that help focus my attention in working with clients include emotional and social intelligence, attachment theory, mentalization, coping style, personal epistemology, and ethical development, among others. My point is not to create a comprehensive list here but to communicate the fact that any theory of human functioning, including all of the developmental theories, are potentially helpful to a holistic therapist. Equally, we can draw on theories of what constitutes a good life and/or contentment from sources outside of the psychological literature. We can look at different forms of philosophy, Eastern psychology, religions, spirituality, etc. To be sure, the techniques and interventions suggested in Psychosynthesis and other forms of holistic therapy are all potentially relevant to our clients' processes.

Besides formal theories we employ in treatment, we are also drawn to address issues and dynamics that have been relevant in past treatments. If I have seen eleven adolescent girls who have experienced incest and with eight of them their relationship with their sister has been an important factor, when client number twelve casually mentions her sister, it will capture my attention. I am likely to ask her to take the conversation in the direction of exploring that relationship. We learn from our clients constantly.

Connection, intention, and attention help us make decisions from moment to moment during therapy. The way that these decisions are communicated—or even if we communicate overtly—is highly important. The work on common factors can be very helpful in this process.

Common Factors

Several researchers have found that there are common approaches to treatment that successful therapists employ, regardless of theoretical commitments. In the Norcross text (2011), there were a number of concrete recommendations for therapists that should be incorporated into any holistic approach to treatment. The primary observation is that the therapist should adapt their relational style to the patient (Norcross and Lambert 2011). This is in keeping with the observation above that connection is the principal piece of a mind-centered approach to holistic psychotherapy. Horvath et al. (2011) found in their review of the literature that "developing a 'good enough' alliance early in therapy is vital for therapy success" (56). They also noted that early in the treatment process, therapists should vary the methods or tasks of treatment in order to find what fits best for the client. Additionally, therapists should not become defensive in response to client negativity or hostility.

In the Norcross volume (2011), Tryon and Winograd (2011, 153-167) discussed the need to work with clients on the goals that the client has identified as important. While most theoretical approaches suggest an ultimate goal for treatment (e.g., to dissolve specific cognitive distortions, to alter unconscious patterns, to reduce the symptoms of a diagnosis, to realize the Self, etc.), successful therapy is premised on the therapist's ability to help the client grow into a position in which they come to realize their own therapeutic endpoint.

Empathy has been found to be the cornerstone of all approaches to therapy. Elliot et al. (2011, 132-152) noted that it is not enough to understand your client; it is crucial that you communicate this understanding. Furthermore, communicating an understanding of experience (mind) rather than simply words is important. These authors found that an important aspect of any kind of therapy is to help clients "deepen their experience and reflexively examine their feelings, values, and goals" (Elliot et al. 2011, 146), which is accomplished by therapists responding to what is not said. The attuned therapist also knows when to express their understanding to the client and when this may feel intrusive or make the client uncomfortable in any way. Not responding to your client is sometimes an important response.

Besides empathy, two other facilitating conditions put forward by Carl Rogers (1957) are, in fact, important for every approach to therapy. Farber and Doolin (2011, 168-186) discussed positive regard, or warm acceptance, and its role in treatment success. The findings confirm that overtly reflecting to the client your honest regard for them as a precious human is crucial for client growth. Likewise, Kolden et al. (2011, 186-202) found that the therapist's congruence or genuineness is an important element in any successful treatment. I have had students note that they believed that being "professional" meant putting some distance between themselves and their clients. If connection is bilateral in treatment, as is a core tenet of a mind-centered approach, how you feel about your client is going to affect the outcome. Sometimes this requires that you engage in a brief compassion exercise before you greet your client. This may be a couple of breaths during which you acknowledge how much pain your client is in and generate a feeling of compassion for your client's suffering.

Other important common factors in treatment include eliciting client feedback on the process of therapy from time to time (Lambert and Shimokawa 2011, 203-223) and repairing the ruptures that are inevitable in treatment (Safran, Muran, and Eubanks-Carter 2011, 224-238). Likewise, regardless of theoretical school, successful therapists are able to successfully manage countertransference (Hayes, Gelso, and Hummel 2011, 239-258). While this construct is most closely associated with Psychodynamic Psychotherapy and Psychoanalysis, its importance transcends theoretical approach. From a mind-centered approach, if there is a true connection between therapist and client and they share an experience of the treatment to some degree, how you feel about your client will be discernible to your client. You will get frustrated. You may get angry or feel hopeless or overwhelmed. Feeling these things is not wrong. Using this information to help your client is an important element of the mind-centered approach to holistic therapy.

The bottom line is that a holistic therapist is well-advised to demonstrate those capacities that are common to all good therapists. If holistic therapy is to move beyond the periphery of bona fide therapies, we must practice high-quality therapy. The research on common factors is a good place to start toward this end.

Interpretation

Several of the holistic approaches to therapy target unconscious processes that are harming the client as well as creating new ways of experiencing that can make life more satisfying for them. In many cases, the therapist has a sense of some of the interfering unconscious patterns or of potential new levels of consciousness that may help the client. The process of sharing such insights with the client is interpretation. Interpretation is the process of offering the client an observation about something that may be operating outside of their awareness (unconsciously). This can be a feeling, or it can be a complex pattern. It can be interactions that they have with others, or it can be a way that they assign meaning to events, including dreams and fantasies. In mind-centered depth therapy, we offer our interpretations tentatively. We ask if it makes sense, if it is helpful, or how it lands. It is possible that when you believe that you have noticed some unconscious process that is operating for the client, your client can reject your observation, saying, "No, it's not like that at all." There are two possibilities here: either you have noted something that may not, in fact, be relevant to this client, or they are not yet ready to confront that particular process. In a mind-centered approach, we do not authoritatively tell our clients what is going on inside of them. We offer observations provisionally, and if they reject our reflection, we accept that it is not helpful now, for whatever reason, and let it go.

When we think we're reflecting back to the client what they just said, we are actually offering an interpretation: "This is the way I heard what you just said. This is what I think it meant." In many cases, our reflection comes as a surprise to the client and reflects something operating outside of their awareness. Reflection often suggests something that the client had been unaware of.

Case Examples

These are some brief excerpts from my holistic approach to therapy. As was emphasized, holistic therapy from a mind-centered perspective is not manualized. Thus, the way the work unfolded in these cases with me is different from the ways they would unfold with you. I offer these cases only to demonstrate how multiple forms of therapy are braided together to help achieve the objectives of mind-centered therapy.

Lisette

Lisette is a woman in her late twenties. She was raised by a single mother who is highly narcissistic. Lisette's reaction to her mother's demands has been to excel. She is a successful professional with an advanced degree.

She suffered for years with polysubstance abuse but has been clean and sober for a year. She also has a history of intense romantic engagements that end in crushing disappointment. In each of her entanglements, she has worked hard to be whatever the object of her desire wants her to be: she believes she wants what they want, and what she thinks she wants changes with each romantic entanglement. If they want to leave the region, she becomes eager to move. If they want to start a small business, she is ready to become an entrepreneur. When one boyfriend wanted to pursue an advanced degree, Lisette applied to doctoral programs. Each time, the relationship ended before she made any life-altering changes.

Lisette is easily emotionally attuned to others. While she feels very deeply for the people in her life, she is quite emotionally restricted when it comes to her own feelings (I suspect this was the role of substance abuse: to regulate repressed affect). She typically presents as quite grounded, quite mature, and quite emotionally controlled. She came in one day after a difficult week at work. We talked about the events of the week and Lisette's responses to those events. As we talked, I wondered if there was some shame operating. Lisette wondered if this was true but did not connect immediately with the idea. I suggested maybe we try a somatic technique to identify if there was anywhere in her body that she was carrying the reaction to the events of the week. She identified her abdomen. Improvising on the Jungian technique of active imagination, I helped Lisette enter a relaxed state (slightly altered state of consciousness or light trance) and give the feeling a symbolic form. As is the case with active imagination, I invited Lisette to carry on a dialogue with the image, to ask what the feeling in her abdomen was trying to communicate, what wisdom it carried. After a few minutes I brought Lisette out of the light trance and invited her to share what she wished about the experience. Lisette identified that the feeling was a big gray boulder but that it wouldn't talk to her. I asked if this seemed familiar. Lisette talked about how when she was a child her mother would not talk to her about difficult feelings. She was not allowed to show any distress around her mother. Her mother would try to stop her expression of feeling and would send her to her room if she did not stop immediately.

Lisette began to cry. Her cries came from her depths, shaking her body. She threw her head back on the couch and sobbed. I told her that the feelings were welcome here, that she was allowed to share her grief and pain in this space. In a purely intuitive moment, I was moved to say, "You're not alone. I'm right here. I'm here."

Lisette cried until she was done. She told me that when I said that Lisette was not alone, she felt nauseous. She felt profoundly how she had always been alone with her difficult feelings. If she showed how she felt, it would be very destructive. I engaged in the mind-centered form of interpretation: "It's like your feelings are dangerous. It's like *you* are dangerous to your mother. You must be banished to your room to protect her." Lisette agreed: "It's a short pipeline from my emotions to *me*."

Lisette said she had never thought of it in this way, but it made sense to her that shame was related to feeling that her emotional response to the difficult week was based on the association that if she had strong feelings, she was dangerous. She needed to stuff those feelings to stay in connection. Being able to feel them and feel that she was not alone while she felt them was transformative for her.

Based on my knowledge of attachment and attunement, I used paralinguistic forms of communication to help Lisette modulate out of her deep grief. That is, I used a lighter, brighter tone as I turned the conversation to more mundane topics so that Lisette could return to baseline functioning and resume her daily routine.

We see here that I used a body-based intervention by identifying where in the body Lisette was experiencing her feelings. In the process of bringing the material into greater awareness, I used a Jungian intervention: active imagination. All of this was undergirded by the intuitive wondering if shame was the foundation of Lisette's reaction to her difficult week. The interpretation was based on me sharing the way the whole narrative made sense to me. It was not offered as the truth but as a possible way to make sense and give meaning to Lisette's experience of her feelings and the overwhelming impact they had on her. In this case, it resonated with Lisette. It offered her an understanding that was meaningful to her. I wonder if Lisette's felt sense that she is dangerous contributes in some way to her becoming whatever her romantic partners want her to be. But like many such thoughts, this one did not come up in treatment. In many cases we engage in silent interpretations: ideas that we file away and may or may not come up later. My point in sharing this is to illustrate that my listening is keyed into possibilities for what my client's unconscious sense of self is, how it came to be that way, and if it is something that the client is ready to confront.

My point in sharing this example is to show that I used more traditional psychotherapeutic interventions from a variety of psychotherapeutic modalities. What unites them is their purpose. In this session, the different interventions were brought to bear on the objective of bringing unconscious feelings into awareness. This required a combination of affect regulation, acceptance, and exploration.

Jennifer

Jennifer is in her early thirties. Her parents were conservative Christians, and she was raised in a hellfire and brimstone environment. She works in a profession that is known to allow verbal abuse. She has been in and out of a relationship with her child's father, who is also verbally abusive. In this case, the therapist postulated that Jennifer has withstood the verbal abuse of her boss, a coworker, and her child's father as a consequence of the verbal abuse her parents engaged in, which they justified by religious doctrines. Much of the focus of the conversation in therapy for several weeks was dominated by an examination of the beliefs Jennifer was taught both in church and in her home in relation to her family's religion.

One of the many ways that Jennifer's early upbringing influenced her sense of self was in relation to body image. She fought to embrace body positivity but typically fell into shame and disgust over her physical appearance. It was very difficult for her to identify as being more than her body. Conversations in therapy included the social categories associated with body shape and how Jennifer's place in that category impacted her sense of self.

An important element in working with the sense of self and body image was to incorporate mindful yoga practice into the treatment. As a variation of Trauma-Sensitive Yoga, I (a certified yoga teacher) helped Jennifer focus on the physical sensations of working, resting, stretching, and contracting muscles along with breathing. The objective here was to help Jennifer feel good in her body and gain a sense of agency over it.

What we see in this case is the relationship between spirituality, social categories, and embodiment in the sense of self. We see the reverberations of spiritual abuse and family abuse on sense of self and how those early childhood experiences set up a pattern that repeated across relationships in adulthood.

Cassandra

Cassandra presented for treatment after a brief hospitalization. She went to the emergency department when she was quite emotionally distraught and suicidal. They stabilized her with medication and suggested therapy. Cassandra was highly emotionally reactive. She was unhappy in her marriage and felt overwhelmed by her preschool daughter. She was also very upset about the current socio-political situation in the US and in the community where she owned a business.

Cassandra was involved in a group of women who were exploring New Age spirituality, although she was not involved in any daily practices like meditation, etc. I led her in some meditation practices and invited Cassandra to continue to experiment with practices she would be comfortable pursuing regularly. She found a meditation app she liked and began to meditate daily. This helped with affect regulation and the ability to access unconscious material.

Once stabilized, I introduced the topic of suicidality with Cassandra. I explored Cassandra's beliefs concerning the soul and what happens before and after death. Cassandra endorsed reincarnation. I encouraged Cassandra to begin to construct a sense of purpose by asking her, "Why are you here now? Why at this historical context?" Cassandra began to identify some important character traits, both those that she wished to nurture and live out and some that brought her guilt and she wished to extinguish. Cassandra began to see her life as meaningful and was looking forward to living with her unique purpose.

Part of the work with this client was integration. Her spirituality, her professionalism, and her family responsibilities and social concerns all seemed to be at odds with each other. We addressed social roles and expectations and how this created strain. We also engaged in a great deal of parts work based on the Internal Family Systems model. As we began to explore various self states and characteristics, Cassandra indicated that she felt herself to be a bully in childhood and continuing through adulthood. She felt a great deal of guilt over the way that she spoke to community members and family. She identified that she had been coercively parented and that she was engaging in coercive parenting. We explored what all of that meant to her. As we deepened in both the parts work and the bullying/coercive parenting, we were inspired to do some shadow work: to look at those parts that she rejected. Cassandra was very interested in pursuing this work with the help of archetype cards, a deck of cards that depict several different archetypal figures with their light aspect and shadow aspect. Being able to integrate many of her self states, including those she had rejected, proved to bring her a great deal of peace and energy.

Discussion

These cases are offered not as the single way to do holistic therapy from a mind-centered perspective but rather illustrate how a mind-centered perspective guides the way that therapists engage with clients—how we begin to conceptualize what might be going on and how we intervene. There is no template or manual. All of therapy becomes an experiment: tell me if this works or not, tell me if this is helpful or not. If so, we keep going in this direction. If not, we'll try something else. The practice is reflective. What we do depends entirely on what just happened.

In all cases, embodiment, spirituality, psychological, social, and, in some cases, energetic considerations are included. How rigidly repeated patterns play out in a person's sense of self, how the social categories and roles affect them, and how their values/character is implicated are important. We are working at all times to integrate unconscious processes and contents and, in many cases, to invite new experiences from the unconscious that are not comprised of a client's personal past, for example, gaining new perspectives in an altered state of consciousness—from the superconscious, if you will.

Conclusion

As a holistic approach to therapy, the mind-centered approach is a reflective practice. We immerse ourselves in the flow of each unique encounter and engage our ability to think and feel our way forward. This process is based on the triumvirate processes of connection, intention, and attention. We must establish a strong connection with clients that is based on fittedness. We choose what and how we discuss with clients, along with any specific techniques we will use, based on that which enhances fittedness. We set our intention to discern and act in a way that responds to what our clients need. We target our attention in this process based on intuition, formal theory, and past clinical experience. This process requires that we are adept at utilizing those relationship capacities that are common to all successful therapy: the common factors. We also use interpretation in a mind-centered approach, but we do so by offering our observations provisionally, we check with our client to see if it is helpful, and we accept the fact that sometimes it is not. We see in these remarks the fact that a mind-centered approach to holistic therapy cannot be codified. It cannot be reduced to formulas or standardized in any way. This does not imply that we "fly be the seat of our pants" but rather that we are centered in and highly knowledgeable about our work.

Holistic Practice Points

- Mind-centered therapy is a reflective approach. Techniques are effective only to the degree they match the needs of a specific client. It is essential that you allow yourself to tune into your own internal processes as you interact with your client and trust the process. As you reflect on what your client is experiencing and how you are experiencing your client, you will arrive at an appropriate response.

- This requires that you form a connection with your client; that you allow your knowledge of formal theory, your intuition, and your past clinical experience to direct your attention to the flow of the session; and that your intention is to allow the client to heal rather than trying to fix them.

- These three features of our work—connection, intention, and attention—produce a healing experience for the client and informs if and when we employ techniques, as well as which ones we may choose to employ.

- Common factors research forms a scaffolding of basic interpersonal capacities all successful therapists must master. The therapeutic alliance, empathy, authenticity, unconditional positive regard, etc. must be at the very center of your work with your client.

- Our work proceeds forward based on connection (or the degree of fittedness we are able to achieve with our client), our intention to work toward our client's healing, and attention.

Chapter Eight

Conclusion

We are educated into a culture in which we have been taught that reality is matter, and that scientism—the view that the scientific method is the only legitimate way to know anything—is true. Thus, when we think about mental suffering, we have difficulty seeing it as something other than a disease of the brain. We have created a mental health system that is based on this medical model. Unfortunately, this approach does not seem to be working too well. Many therapists have suggested that looking beyond the biological aspects of humanity and approaching mental wellness from a holistic perspective can produce more profound long-lasting relief from mental strife.

But what is holistic psychotherapy? Is it anything that throws in an intervention that is not talk therapy? As we reviewed the various approaches to treatment that self-identify as holistic, we came to see several important areas of overlap. Perhaps primarily, holistic therapy is not bio-reductionist. Biology is an important aspect of being human. Our bodies and our minds are correlated to a very high degree. But mental healing must transcend biological interventions.

Like biology, spirituality is fundamental to well-being. After all, psyche means both mind and spirit. But we need to be sensitive to the fact that spirituality is not restricted to religion. Spirituality is a way of making meaning, and certainly various philosophical systems help people in this endeavor. Interventions from Western, Eastern, and Indigenous worldviews can be very helpful in a holistic approach to therapy. But in and of themselves, they are not sufficient in making therapy holistic.

Psychological considerations are perhaps an obvious aspect of holistic psychotherapy. But we must understand that the human mind is not an isolated phenomenon that exists within one's head or even body. Psychological considerations mean we look at all psychological functions, including thought, emotions, intuition, perceptions, and, perhaps most importantly, the sense of self.

The social aspects of self should be equally centered in any holistic approach to therapy. We must help people understand the damaging ways that society prevents them from being the best version of themselves. We must take to heart the fact that while our clients are individuals and must be appreciated as such, they are also connected to everything else that exists. It is the twin attributes of self, both individual and connected, that must be integrated in a successful holistic therapy.

Holistic therapy must also consider the possible role of energy in healing. There is a growing body of literature on energy healing and the role of energy in suffering and well-being. Eastern and Indigenous healing systems place energy at the center of their understanding of humanity. We must consider that these perspectives have a good deal to teach us about helping people overcome mental suffering and combine this information with our Western knowledge.

Besides being psycho-social-spiritual-energetic-biological, holistic therapy calls on an understanding of what it means to be human and what it means to live a good life well beyond a single discipline. We look at multiple disciplines, and we look at humanity from the perspectives of non-Western people. We acknowledge the wisdom of interventions and techniques that go beyond talk therapy even while acknowledging that talk therapy is a powerful tool.

Using these multiple lenses is still not sufficient to make an approach holistic. We must bring each individual piece together by an overarching logic or metatheory. If holistic psychotherapy is to be anything other than a hodgepodge of this and that, we must understand the why of what we're doing. Psychosynthesis, Integral Therapy, and mind-centered therapy all converge on the metatheoretical perspective that everything is One and that integration is fundamental to well-being.

These three holistic approaches also converge on the idea that mind can be viewed as a heuristic having different levels. They all support work that is aimed at the subconscious, meaning that there is material particular to an individual and their life histories of which they are unaware. There is also superconsciousness, or the potential for transpersonal experiences or to experience in a completely new way. Bringing the nonconscious into awareness is important in this work. Integrating the different forms of consciousness is a requirement for well-being.

All three models place the self at the center of treatment focus. The models differ on the role of normative developmental lines in problems in living. For Assagioli ([1965] 2012) and Chaudhuri ([1968] 1975) as well as in mind-centered depth therapy, individuals must be seen as unique, living individualized developmental arcs. For Wilber (2000) and Foreman (2010), deviation from normative developmental lines is at the root of psychological suffering. Both systems see spiritual realization as the epitome of mental health. Assagioli places less emphasis on the social contribution to suffering than does Sri Aurobindo (McDermont2001).

The three approaches to holistic therapy differ in terms of the degree to which the practice can be codified. Mind-centered depth therapy, like Psychosynthesis, insists that treatment cannot be manualized. It is a reflective practice that unfolds based on connection, intention, and attention. Attention requires that we are versed in a number of formal theories of what constitutes a good life, on our intuition, and on our practice wisdom. This system of treatment requires that one be adept at the common factors that are bedrock for all systems of therapy. It also recognizes that interpretation can be a very valuable tool, though we must be humble in offering any insight to our clients.

The stereotype for holistic therapists is "woo-woo." There seems to be a sense that we fly by the seat of our pants and have no sense of direction or purpose, blithely ignoring the vast literature on psychotherapy. Indeed, we may place very little weight on outcome studies, but this is based on an understanding of the world and human well-being that is complex, cohesive, and coherent. To be adept at this approach to therapy, the clinician must have a breadth of understanding about the human condition. We equally trust our intuition and clinical judgment as important elements in the art form we call therapy. We apply this art to help people heal, and we trust that in doing so, we are contributing to the healing of the social order and the planet. Lofty goals indeed.

References

Alvarez, Anna S., Marco Pagani, and Paolo Meucci. 2012. "The Clinical Application of the Biopsychosocial Model in Mental Health." *The American Journal of Physical Medicine and Rehabilitation* 91, no. 13 (Suppl. 1): S173-S180. doi: 10.1097/PHM.0b013e31823d54be.

American Society for Psychical Research. "About the society." http://www.aspr.com/who.htm. Accessed 12/4/23.

Arnd-Caddigan, Margaret. *Intuition in Therapeutic Practice: A Mind-Centered Depth Approach for Healing.* London: Routledge, 2021.

Aron, Lewis. 1990. "One Person and Two Person Psychologies and the Method of Psychoanalysis." *Psychoanalytic Psychology* 7 (4): 475-485.

Assagioli, Roberto. (1965) 2012. *Psychosynthesis: A collection of basic writings.* Amherst, MA: Synthesis Center. Page numbers are from the Synthesis Center edition.

Asthana, H. S. 2015. "Wilhem Wundt." *Psychology Studies* 6 (2): 244-248.

Audate, Terry S. 2022. "Psychosynthesis as a Spiritual Practice in Clinical Social Work." *Journal of Religion and Spirituality in Social Work: Social Thought* 41 (4): 369-383. doi: 10.1080/15426432.2022.2103060.

Banerji, Debashish. 2012. "Structure and Process: Integral Philosophy and Triple Transformation." *Integral Review* 8 (1): 85-95.

Baruss, Imants and Julia Mossbridge. 2017. *Transcendent Mind: Rethinking the Science of Consciousness.* Washington, D.C.: American Psychological Association.

Bass, Anthony. 2015. "The Dialogue of Unconsciousness, Mutual Analysis and the Use of Self in Contemporary Relational Psychoanalysis." *Psychoanalytic Dialogues* 25 (1): 2-17.

Bauer, Susan W. 2015. *The story of Western Science: From the Writings of Aristotle to the Big Bang Theory.* New York: W.W. Norton.

Barford, Duncan, Filip Geerardyn, and Vijver van der Gertusvan. 2002. *The Pre-Psychoanalytic Writings of Sigmund Freud.* London: Routledge.

Ben-Shahar, Asaf R. 2012. "Do Cry for Me Argentina! The Challenges Trauma Work Poses for Holistic Psychotherapy." *Movement and Dance in Psychotherapy* 7 (1): 7-21. doi: 10.1080/17432979.2011.629100.

Blumer, Herbert. 1969. *Symbolic Interactionism: Perspective and Method.* Englewood Cliffs, NJ: Prentice-Hall, Inc.

Boston Change Process Study Group. 2010. *Change in Psychotherapy: A Unifying Paradigm.* New York: W.W. Norton.

Brabrant, Oliver. 2016. "More Than Meets the Eye: Towards a Post-Materialist Model of Consciousness." *Explore: The Journal of Science and Healing* 12, no. 5 (Sept.-Oct.): 347-354. https://doi.org/10.1016/j.explore.2016.06.006.

Brown, Molly Y. 2022. "Psychosynthesis and Humanity's Turning." In *Know, Love, Transform Yourself: Theory, Techniques and New Developments in Psychosynthesis (Vol. 2)*, edited by Petra G. Nocelli, 421-432. n.p.: Psychosynthesis Books.

Bruce, Steve. 2020. *British Gods: Religion in Modern Britain.* Oxford: Oxford University Press.

Burbank, Patricia M., and Diane C. Martins. 2009. "Symbolic Interactionism and Critical Perspective: Divergent or Synergistic?" *Nursing Philosophy* 11 (1): 25–41. doi.org/10.1111/j.1466-769X.2009.00421.x.

Burke, Peter J. and Jan E. Stets. 2023. *Identity Theory: Revised and Expanded.* 2 ed.. Oxford: Oxford University Press.

Campbell, James. 2017. *Experiencing William James: Belief in a Pluralistic World.* Charlottesville VA: University of Virginia Press.

Carter, Michael. J. and Celene Fuller. 2015. "Symbolic interactionism." *Sociopedia.isa.* doi: 10.1177/205684601561.

Carveth, Donald. L. 2012. "Concordant and Complementary Countertransference: A Clarification." In *Psychoanalytic Thinking: A Dialectical Critique of Contemporary Theory and Practice,* edited by Donald L. Carveth, 168-180. London: Routledge.

Chalmers, David. 1995. "Facing up to the Problem of Consciousness." https://consc.net/papers/facing.pdf. 1-27. Accessed 11/13/23.

Chaudhuri, Haridas. (1965) 2019. *Integral yoga: The Concept of Harmonious and Creative Living*. London: Routledge. Page numbers are from the Routledge edition.

Chaudhuri, Haridas. (1968) 1975. *Mastering the Problems of Living*. Wheaton, IL: Quest. Page numbers are from the Quest edition.

Cornelissen, Matthijs. 2018. "The Self and the Structure of the Personality: An Overview of Sri Aurobindo's Topography of Consciousness. *International Journal of Transpersonal Studies* 37 (1): 63-89.

Cortright, Brant. 2007. *Integral psychology: Yoga, growth, and opening the heart*. New York: State University of New York Press.

Damasio, Antonio. 1994. *Descartes' Error: Emotion, Reason, and the Human Brain*. New York: Quill.

Damien, Rodica I., Marion Spengler, Andreea Sutu, and Brent W. Roberts, 2018. "Sixteen Going on Sixty: A Longitudinal Study of Personality Stability and Change Across 50 Years." *Journal of Personality and Social Psychology* 117 (3): doi:: 10.1037/pspp0000210.

Dein, Simon. 2010. "Judeo-Christian Religious Experiences and Psychopathology: The Legacy of William James. *Transcultural Psychiatry*, 47 (4): 523-547. doi: 10.1177/1363461510377568.

Devonis, David C. 2014. *History of Psychology 101*. Ann Arbor, MI: Springer.

Duignan, Brian. 2018. "Plato and Aristotle: How Do They Differ?." *Encyclopedia Britannica*. https://www.britannica.com/story/plato-and-aristotle-how-do-they-differ Accessed 11/12/23.

Duncan, Barry L, Scott D. Miller, Bruce E. Wampold, and Mark A. Hubble (Eds). 2010. *The Heart and Soul of Change: Delivering What Works in Therapy* 2 ed. Washington, D.C.: American Psychological Association.

Duncan, Barry. 2010. "Prologue: Saul Rosenzweig: The Gounder of Common Factors." In *The Heart and Soul of Change: Delivering What Works in Therapy* 2 ed., edited by Barry L. Duncan, Scott D. Miller, Bruce E. Wampold, and Mark A. Hubble, 3-22. Washington, D. C.: American Psychological Association.

Duval, James, Kevin Clouthier, and Gary Dumbrill. 1999. "All Have Won, Therefore, All Deserve Prizes: An Interview with Scott Miller." *Journal of Systemic Therapies* 18 (3): 77-93.

Easton, Mark. 2022. "Cosmic Consciousness: William James, Henry James and the Society for Psychical Research." In *Science and Religion in Western Literature: Critical Theological Studies,* edited by Michael Fuller, 110-125. London: Routledge.

Edge, Linda. W. 2011. *The Eclectic Practitioner: Becoming Holistic.* n.p.: KT Press.

Elkins, David. N. 2005. "A Humanistic Approach to Spiritually Oriented Psychotherapy." In *Spiritually Oriented Psychotherapy, edited by Len Sperry and Edward P.* Sharansky, 131–151. Washington, D.C.: American Psychological Association.

Elliott, Robert, Arthur C. Bohart, Jeanne C. Watson, and Leslie S. Greenberg. 2011. "Empathy." In *Psychotherapy Relationships That Work: Evidence-Based Responsiveness.* 2 ed., edited by. John C. Norcross, 132-152. Oxford: Oxford University Press.

Ellis, Albert. 1962. *Reason and Emotion in Psychotherapy.* New York: Stuart.

Emerson, David. 2015. *Trauma Sensitive Yoga in Therapy: Bringing the Body into Treatment.* New York: W.W. Norton.

Extremera, Natalio and Pablo Fernandez-Berrocal. 2006. "Emotional Intelligence as Predictor of Mental, Social, and Physical Health in University Students." *The Spanish Journal of Psychology* 9 (1): 45-51.

Farber, Barry A., and Erin M. Doolin. 2011. Positive Regard and Affirmation. In *Psychotherapy Relationships That Work: Evidence-Based Responsiveness* 2 ed., edited by John. C. Norcross, 168-186. Oxford: Oxford University Press.

Forman, Mark. D. 2010. *A guide to Integral Psychotherapy: Complexity, Integration, and Spirituality in Practice.* Albany, NY: SUNY Press.

Fonagy, Peter, Gyorgy Gergely, Elliot Jurist, and Mary Target. 2005. *Affect Regulation, Mentalization, and the Development of the Self.* New York: Other Press.

Frank, Jerome. D. and Julia D. Frank. 1973. *Persuasion and Healing: A Comparative Study of Psychotherapy.* Baltimore: Johns Hopkins University.

Freud, Sigmund. 2004. *The Unconscious.* Modern Penguin Classics. London: Penguin Classics.

Ghose, Aurobindo. 2001. "The Sevenfold Chord of Being." In *The Essential Aurobindo: Writings of Sri Aurobindo,* edited by Robert McDermott, 83-91. Herdon, VA: Lindisfarne Books.

Gilligan, Carol. 1982. *In a Different Voice: Psychological Theory and Women's Development.* Cambridge, MA: Harvard University Press.

Goodrick-Clarke, Nicholas. 2008. *The Western Esoteric Traditions: A Historical Introduction.* Oxford: Oxford University Press.

Graubard, Rachel, Ariadna Perez-Sanchez, and Rajani Katta. 2021. "Stress and Skin: An Overview of Mind Body Therapies as a Treatment Strategy in Dermatology." *Dermatology Practice Concepts* 11 (4): doi: 10.5826/dpc.1104a91. PMID: 34631261; PMCID: PMC8480446.

Grossman, Lee. 2023. *The Psychoanalytic Encounter and the Misuse of Theory.* London: Routledge.

Haidt, Jonathan, Fredrik Björklund, and Scott Murphy. 2000. "Moral Dumbfounding: When Intuition Finds No Reason." https://polpsy.ca/wp-content/uploads/2019/05/haidt.bjorklund.pdf. Accessed 1/3/24.

Haimovich, Saul. 2002. "Freud's Pre-Analytical Writings and His Scientific Revolution. In *The pre-psychoanalytic writings of Sigmund Freud,* edited by Duncan Barford, Filip Geerardyn, and Gertrudis van de Vijver, 207-214. London: Routledge.

Hakomi Institute. n.d. "Principles." https://hakomiinstitute.com/about/hakomi-mindful-somatic-psychotherapy/the-hakomi-principles. Accessed 12/20/23.

Hayes, R. A. 2004. "Introduction to Evidence-Based Practices." In *The Evidence-Based Practice: Methods, models, and Tools for Mental Health Professionals,* edited by Chris E. Stout and Randy A. Hayes, 1-9. Hoboken, N.J.: John Wiley and Sons.

Hayes, Jeffrey A., Charles J. Gelso, and Ann M. Hummel. 2011 "Managing countertransference." In *Psychotherapy Relationships That Work: Evidence-Based Responsiveness.* 2 ed., edited by John C. Norcross, 239-258. Oxford: Oxford University Press.

Heineman, Martha. B. 1981. "The Obsolete Scientific Imperative in Social Work Research." *Social Service Review* 55 (3): 371-397.

Herman, 2018. "Integral Psychology." *International Journal of Transpersonal Studies* 37 (1): 245-249.

Holmes, J. 2000. "Narrative in Psychiatry and Psychotherapy: The Evidence?" *Journal of Medical Ethics* 26: 92-96.

Horvath, Adam O., A. C. Del Re, Christopher Fluckiger, and Dianne Symonds. 2011. "Alliance in Individual Psychotherapy." In *Psychotherapy Relationships That Work: Evidence-Based Responsiveness.* 2 ed., edited by John C. Norcross, 25-69. Oxford: Oxford University Press.

Hunt, Morton. 2007. *The Story of Psychology.* New York: Anchor Books.

Hutton, Ronald. 2019. *The Triumph of the Moon: A History of Modern Pagan Witchcraft.* Oxford: Oxford University Press.

Insel, Thomas. 2022. *Healing: Our path from mental illness to mental health.* London: Penguin.

Jacobs GD. 2001a. "Clinical Applications of the Relaxation Response and Mind-Body Interventions." *Journal of Alternative Complementary Medicine* 7, (Supp 1): S93-doi: 10.1089/107555301753393850. 101.

Jacobs, G.D. 2001b. "The Physiology of Mind-Body Interactions: The Stress Response and the Relaxation Response. *Journal of Alternative and Complementary Medicine* 7, (Suppl. 1): 83-92. doi: 10.1089/107555301753393841.

James, William. 1958. *The varieties of religious experience: A study in human nature.* Dublin: Mentor.

Jurist, Elliot. 2019. *Minding Emotions: Cultivating Mentalization in Psychotherapy.* New York: Guilford Press.

Keppler, Joachim and Itay Shani. 2020. "Cosmopsychism and Consciousness Research: A Fresh View on the Causal Mechanisms Underlying Phenomenal States. *Frontiers in Psychology* 11: 1-7. https://doi.org/10.3389/fpsyg.2020.00371.

Kihlstrom, J.F. 1999. "The psychological unconscious." In *Handbook of Personality: Theory and Research.* 2 ed., edited by Lawrence. A. Pervin and Oliver P. John, 424–442. New York: Guilford Press.

Koldin, Gregory G., Marjorie H. Klein, Chia-Chiang Wang, and Sara B. Austin. 2011. "Congruence/Genuineness." In *Psychotherapy Relationships That Work: Evidence-Based Responsiveness.* 2 ed., edited by John C. Norcross, 186-202. Oxford: Oxford University Press.

Kurtz, Ron. 1990. *Body-Centered Psychotherapy: The Hakomi Method.* Coopersburg, PA: LifeRhythm.

Lakoff, George. 1988. "Cognitive Semantics." In *Meaning and Mental Representations,* edited by Umberto Eco, Marco Santambriogio, and Patrizia Violi, 119-153. Bloomington: Indiana University Press.

Lambert, Michael. J. and Kenichi Shimokawa. 2011. Collecting Client Feedback. In *Psychotherapy Relationships That Work: Evidence-Based Responsiveness* 2 ed., edited by John C. Norcross, 203-223. Oxford: Oxford University Press.

Lebow, Jay. L. and Paul H. Jenkins. 2018. *Research for the Psychotherapist: From Science to Practice.* London: Routledge.

Lee, M.S., M.H. Pittler, and E. Ernst. 2008. "Effects of Reiki in Clinical Practice." *International Journal of Clinical Practice* 62 (6): 10.1111/j.1742-1241.2008.01729.x

Lilienfeld, Scott O, and Hal Arkowitz. 2012. "Are All Psychotherapies Created Equal?" *Scientific American*: https://www.scientificamerican.com/article/are-all-psychotherapies-created-equal/. Accessed 10/10/23.

Loizzo, Josehp. 2023. "Introduction." In *Advances in Contemplative Psychotherapy: Accelerating Personal and Social Transformation,* edited by Joseph Loizzo, Fiona Brandon, Emily J. Wolf, and Miles Neale, xxv-xlii. London: Routledge.

LynLake Centers for Wellbeing. "Somatic experiencing: A body-centered for treating PTSD." https://therapy-mn.com/blog/somatic-experiencing-ptsd/#:~:text=Somatic%20Experiencing%20is%20a%20body,conceptualized%20by%20trauma%20therapist%20Dr. Accessed 1/4/24.

Main, Roderick. 2006. "Religion." In *The handbook of Jungian Psychology: Theory ,Practice, and Applications,* edited by Renos K. Papadopoulos, 296-323 London: Routledge.

Marsonet, Michele. 2019. "Philosophy and Logical Positivism." *Academicus International Scientific Journal* 10 (19): 32-36.

Majied, Kamilah. 2023. "Contemplative Practices for Assessing and Eliminating Racism in Psychotherapy." In *Advances in Contemplative Psychotherapy: Accelerating Personal and Social Transformation* 2 ed., edited by Joseph Loizzo, Fiona Brandon, Emily J. Wolf, and Miles Neale, 3-12. London: Routledge.

Mayden, Kelley. D. 2012. "Mind-Body Therapies: Evidence and Implications in Advanced Oncology Practice. *Journal of Advanced Practice in Oncology 3*: 357-373.

Mazzotta, Laura, ed. 2022. *Holistic Mental Health: Calm, Clear, and in Control for the Rest of your Life.* Bethesda, MD: Brave Healer Productions.

McDermott, Robert A., ed. *The Essential Aurobindo: Writings of Sri Aurobindo.* Herdon, MA.: Lindisfarne Books.

Medhananda, Swami. 2021. "Cutting the Knot of the World Problem: Sri Aurobindo's Experiential and Philosophical Critique of Advaita Vedanta." *Religions* 12 (9): 1-21. https:// doi.org/10.3390/ rel1290765. Doi.org/10.24972/ijts/2018.37.1.120.

Medhananda, Swami. 2022. "The Playful Self-Involution of Divine Consciousness: Sri Aurobindo's Evolutionary Cosmopsychism and His Response to the Individuation Problem." *The Monist* 105 (1): 92-109.

Moffatt, Kelsey M., Holly K. Oxhandler, and James W. Ellor. 2021. "Religion and Spirituality in Graduate Social Work Education: A National Survey." *Journal of Social Work Education* 57 (2): 287-29. doi: 10.1080/10437797.2019.1670307.

National Institutes of Health National Center for Complimentary and Integrative Health. "Mind and Body Practices. https://www.nccih.nih.gov/health/mind-and-body-practices. Accessed 12/20/23.

Nelson, Katherine. 1985. *Making Sense: The Acquisition of Shared Meaning*. New York: Academic Press.

Nocelli, Petra G. 2021. *Know, Love, Transform Yourself. Theory, Techniques and New Developments in Psychosynthesis Vol. 1*. n.p.: Psychosynthesis Books.

Nocelli, Petra. G. 2022. *Know, Love, Transform Yourself. Theory, Techniques and New Developments in Psychosynthesis Vol. II*. n.p.: Psychosynthesis Books.

Norcross, John. C., ed. 2011. *Psychotherapy Relationships that Work: Evidence-Based Responsiveness*. 2 ed. Oxford: Oxford University Press.

Norcross, John C. and Michael J. Lambert. 2011. "Evidence-Based Therapy Relationships." In P*sychotherapy Relationships That Work: Evidence-Based Responsiveness* 2 ed., edited by John C. Norcross, 3-24. Oxford: Oxford University Press.

Nungesser, Frithjof. 2021. "Pragmatism and Interaction." In *The Routledge Handbook of Interactionism*, edited by Dirk vom Lehn, Nataila Ruiz-Junco, and Will Gibson, 25- 36. London: Routledge.

Pargament, Kenneth I. and Stephen M. Saunders. 2007. "Introduction to the Special Issue on Spirituality and Psychotherapy. *Psychology Faculty Research and Publication* 310. https://epublications.marquette.edu/psych_fac/310

PDM Task Force. 2006. *Psychodynamic Diagnostic Manual*. Silver Spring, MD: Alliance of Psychoanalytic Organizations.

Porges, Stephen. W. 2022. "Polyvagal Theory: A Science of Safety." *Frontiers in Integrative Neuroscience* 16 (871227): 1-15. doi: 10.3389/fnint.2022.871227.

Psychiatry.org. n.d. DSM history. psychiatry.org/psychiatrists/practice/dsm/about-dsm/history-of-the-dsm. Accessed 9/12/23.

Quirke, Viviane and Jon-Paul Gaudillière. 2008. "The Era of Biomedicine: Science, Medicine, and Public Health in Britain and France after the Second World War. *Medical History* 52 (4): 41-52. doi: 10.1017/s002572730000017x.

Racker, Heinrich. 1957. "The Meanings and Uses of Countertransference." *Psychoanalytic Quartherly* 76 (3): 725-777.

Remizid, Donata. 2012. "The Vienna Circle's 'Scientific World-Conception': Philosophy of Science in the Political Arena." *HOPOS: The Journal of the International Society for the History of Philosophy of Science* 2 (2): 205-242.

Rhine Online. What is Parapsychology?" https://www.rhineonline.org/what-is-parapsychology. Accessed 11/24/23.

Rhodes, Phillip., William Archibald Thomson, Robson, Robert G. Richardson, E. Ashworth Underwood, and Douglas James Guthrie. December 5, 2023. "History of Medicine." *Encyclopedia Britannica.* https://www.britannica.com/science/history-of-medicine.

Rogers, Carl R. 1957. "The Necessary and Sufficient Conditions of Therapeutic Change." *Journal of Consulting Psychology 21 (2)*: 95–103. https://doi.org/10.1037/h0045357.

Saad, Marcelo, and Roberta de Medeiros. 2020. "Advocating for the Concept of Spiritual Health. *American Journal of Emergency Medicine* 45: 563-564. doi: 10.1016/j.ajem.2020.11.080.

Safran, Jeffrey D., J. Christopher Muran, and Catherine Eubanks-Carter. 2011. "Repairing Alliance Ruptures." In *Psychotherapy Relationships That Work: Evidence-Based Responsiveness.* 2 ed., edited by John C. Norcross, 224-238. Oxford: Oxford University Press.

Salvini, Franco. 2022. "Awareness of the Body, Awareness of the Soul. In *Know, Love, Transform Yourself: Theory, Techniques and New Developments in Psychosynthesis (Vol. II)*, edited by Petra Nocelli, 321-339. n.p. Psychosynthesis Books.

Schlitz, Marilyn, Dean Radin, Bertram F. Malle, Stefan Schmidt, Jessica Utts and Garret L. Yount. 2003. "Distant Healing Intention: Definitions and Evolving Guidelines for Laboratory Studies." *Alternative Therapies in Health and Medicine* 9 (3): A31-43.

Schmidt, Stefan. 2015. "Experimental Research on Distant Intention Phenomena." In *Parapsychology, a Handbook for the 21ˢᵗ Century,* edited by Etzel Cardena, J. Palmer, and D. Marcusson-Clavertz 244-257. Jefferson, NC: McFarland and Co.

Schon, Donald. A. 1984. *The Reflective Practitioner: How Professionals Think in Action.* New York: Basic Books.

Schwartz, Ricard. C. and Martha Sweezy. 2019. *Internal Family Systems.* 2 ed. New York: Guilford Press.

Segal, Hanna. 1992. "Countertransference." In *Countertransference: Theory, Technique, Teaching,* edited by Athena Alexandris and Grigoris Vaslamatzis. 13-20. London: Routledge.

Sensorimotor Psychotherapy Institute. https://sensorimotorpsychotherapy.org/about/. Accessed 11/3/23.

Shiah, Yung-Jong, Liang Shan, Dean I. Radin and George T-J Huang. 2022. "Effects of Intentionally Treated Water on the Growth of Mesenchymal Stem Cells: An Exploratory Study." *Explore* 18 (6): 663-669.

Shirazi, Bahnam. 2018. "Haridas Chaudhuri's Contributions to Integral Psychology." *International Journal of Transpersonal Studies* 37 (1): 55-62.

Simmons, Daniel. J. and Christopher F. Chabris. 1999. "Gorillas in Our Midst: Sustained Inattentional Blindness for Dynamic Events." *Perceptions* 28: 1059-1074.

Slade, Darren. M., Adrianna Smell, Elizabeth Wilson, and Rebekah Drumston. 2023. "Percentage of U. S. Adults Suffering from Religious Trauma." *Socio-Historical Examination of Religion and Ministry* 5, no.1: 1-28. doi:10.33929/sherm.2023.vol5.no1.01.

Sorensen, Kenneth. 2016. *The soul of Psychosynthesis: The Seven Core Concepts.* n.p.: Kentaur, 2016.

Stern, Daniel. 2005. "Intersubjectivity." In *The American Psychiatric Publishing Textbook of Psychoanalysis,* edited by Ethel S. Person, Arnold M. Cooper, and Glenn O. Gabbard, 77–92. American Psychiatric Publishing, Inc.

Stern, Steven. 2017. *Needed Relationships and Psychoanalytic Healing: A Holistic Relational Perspective on the Therapeutic Process.* London: Routledge.

Strawson, Galen. 2017. *The Subject of Experience.* Oxford: Oxford University Press.

Stickle, Marilyn. and Margaret Arnd-Caddigan. 2019. *Intuition in Psychotherapy: From Research to Practice.* London: Routledge.

Stricker, G. 2021. "An Introduction to Psychotherapy Integration." *Psychiatric Times* 18, no. 7 (July 1): https://www.psychiatrictimes.com/view/introduction-psychotherapy-integration.

Sur, Roger L., and Philipp Dahm. 2011. "History of Evidence-Based Medicine." *Indian Journal of Neurology* 27 (4): https://journals.lww.com/indianjurol/fulltext/2011/27040/history_of_evidence_based_medicine.11.aspx.

Suris, Alina, Ryan Holliday, and Carol S. North. 2016: "The Evolution of the Classification of Psychiatric Disorders." *Behavioral Sciences* 6 (5): doi:10.3390/bs6010005

Thompson, Neil. 2019. *Mental health and well-being: Alternatives to the Medical Model.* London: Routledge.

Thompson, Neil. 2020. "Mental Health Problems: Getting to the HEART of Resilience." In *Promoting Resilience: Responding to Adversity, Vulnerability, and Loss,* edited by Neil Thompson and Gerry. R. Cox, 64-71. London: Routledge.

Tronick, Edward Z., Nadia Bruschweiler-Stern, Alexadra M. Harrison, Karlen Lyons-Ruth, Alexander C. Morgan, Jeremy P. Nahum, Louis Sander, and Stern, Daniel. N. 1999. "Dyadically Expanded States of Consciousness and Therapeutic Change." *Infant Mental Health Journal* 19 (3): 290-299.

Tryon, Georiana Shick and Greta Winograd. 2011. "Goal Consensus and Collaboration. In *Psychotherapy Relationships That Work: Evidence-Based Responsiveness* 2 ed., edited by John C. Norcross. 153-167. Oxford: Oxford University Press.

Uibel, Thomas. 2022. "Vienna Circle." *The Stanford Encyclopedia of Philosophy*, *edited by* Edward N. Zalta and Uri Nodelman. URL = 98-<https://plato.stanford.edu/archives/fall2022/entries/vienna-circle/>.

University of Cambridge. "Society for Psychical Research." https://www.lib.cam.ac.uk/collections/departments/archives-modern-and-medieval-manuscripts-and-university-archives-0. Accessed11/2/23

Van Strien, Marij. 2022. "The Vienna Circle Against Quantum Speculations." *HOPOS: The Journal of the International Society for the History of Philosophy of Science* 12 (2): 359-394.

Ventriglio, Antonio., Julio Torales, and Disesh Bughra. 2017. "Disease Versus Illness: What Do Clinicians Need to Know?" *International Journal of Social Psychiatry* 63 (1): 3–4. doi: 10.1177/0020764016658677.

Verhaeghe, Paul. 2004. *On being Normal and Other Disorders*. London: Routledge.

Verywellmind.com. "Is Holistic Therapy Right for You?" Last modified on Nov. 21, 2023. https://www.verywellmind.com/holistic-therapy-definition-types-techniques-and-efficacy-5196420.

Vieten, Cassandra and Shelly Scammell. 2015. *Spiritual and Religious Competencies in Clinical Practice: Guidelines for Psychotherapists and Mental Health Professionals*. Oakland, CA: New Harbinger Publications.

Vogel, Michael. J., Mark R. McMinn, Mary A. Peterson, and Kathleen Gathercoal. 2013. "Examining Religion and Spirituality as Diversity Training: A Multidimensional Look at Training in the American Psychological Association." *Professional Psychology: Research and Practice* 44 (3): 158-167.

Wampold, Bruce E. (2010). "The Research Evidence for Common Factor Models: A Historically Situated Perspective. In *The Heart and Soul of Change: Delivering What Works in Therapy* 2 ed., edited by Barry Duncan, Scott D. Miller, Bruce E. Wampold, and Mark A. Hubble. 49-81. Washington, D.C.: American Psychological Association.

Warner, John. H. 1995. "The History of Science and the Sciences of Medicine." *Osiris* 10: 164-193.

White, Kate. 2014. *How do we Integrate Working with the Body in Psychotherapy from an Attachment Perspective?* London: Routledge.

Wilber, Ken. 2000. *Integral Psychology: Consciousness, Spirit, Psychology, Therapy.* Boulder, CO: Shambala.

Winkielman, Piotr. and Kent C. Berridge. 2004. "Unconscious Emotion." *Current Directions in Psychological Science* 13 (3): 120-123.

Zahourak, Rothlyn. P. 2020. "Theory: Intentionality in the Matrix of Healing: A Theory Revised with Non-Nurse Care Practitioners." *Journal of Holistic Nursing* 38 (3): 287-299.

Zarbo, Cristina, Giorgio A. Tasca, Francesco Cattafi, and Angelo Compare. 2015. "Integrative Psychotherapy Works." *Fronters in Psychology* 6: 1-3. doi: 10.3389/fpsyg.2015.02021.

About the Author

Dr. Arnd-Caddigan is a retired faculty member at East Carolina University. She has taught, researched, and practiced psychotherapy for many years. Her life-work has been learning why mental suffering is so widespread in our world today and finding ways to help people heal.

Prior to earning her doctorate in Clinical Social Work, Dr. Arnd-Caddigan studied the history of religions. The knowledge she gained in this process has spurred her to investigate non-Western and holistic approaches to the mind. She strongly believes that if we are going to help people find a way out of mental suffering, we must take a new approach to understanding the mind.

In her retirement from academia, Dr. Arnd-Caddigan runs the Institute for Mind-Centered Therapy PLLC where she conducts therapy, supervision, consultation, and continuing education.

www.ingramcontent.com/pod-product-compliance
Lightning Source LLC
Chambersburg PA
CBHW061534120726
48001CB00004B/1540